PRAISE FOR *FINDING THE RIGHT PSYCHIATRIST*

"Dr. Taylor's book bursts at the seams with insights, study results, and clear-headed explanations. If you are thinking of seeing a psychiatrist, there is no better guide on the market."—Daniel Carlat, assoc. clinical professor of psychiatry, Tufts School of Medicine

"Taylor delineates what's wrong with mental health care today, and guides the reader to that rare psychiatrist who embodies what psychiatric care is—or should be—all about."—Steve Balt, M.D., M.S., Editor-in-Chief, *The Carlat Psychiatry Report*

"I recommend it with enthusiasm! It reads very well, as a comfortable, wise friend talking to you. Practical and reader-friendly covering topics from ADHD, depression, and alternate drugs, to understanding personality, discussing useful techniques in psychotherapy, and creating windows into the mind."—E. Fuller Torrey, M.D., The Stanley Medical Research Institute, and author of *Surviving Schizophrenia*

"An instructive, easy-to-read, insider's view of what to look for in a good psychiatrist and how to avoid an overreliance on diagnoses and psychodrugs that loses your mind."—Mark Ragins, M.D., Psychiatrist, Mental Health America of Los Angeles-Village

"If I were in need of a psychiatrist, I would read this book and heed its advice. Physicians training to be psychiatrists should read it too." —Robert Whitaker, author of *Anatomy of an Epidemic*

"Understanding psychiatric disorders is extremely complex. Accessing appropriate and effective treatment is complicated. Dr. Taylor's book educates individuals living with psychiatric disorders how to search for qualified, effective psychiatric care."—Gary L. Mihelish, D.M.D., NAMI, National Board of Directors

"Provides a plethora of insights in a teaching modality, helping understand strengths and weaknesses of American psychiatry. A much needed resource to educate the public about misdiagnosis and overuse of drugs."—Suzon Kemp, Mental Health Association of Texas Board Member (ret.)

"Dr. Taylor's insightful analysis of how modern mental health care has become a compartmentalized splintered system is a knowledgeable resource for patients and professionals in the challenging times ahead."—Patrick L. Wayne, Consumer Advocate, Community Outreach Specialist, State of Montana

"Taylor is lucid and fearless [in] describing the current state of psychiatry and what he sees as its coming diminished status as a medical specialty. *Finding the Right Psychiatrist* [...] merits the serious attention of psychiatrists who wish to learn how [...] they might practice authentically in spite of this limiting condition."—René J. Muller, Ph.D., author of *Doing Psychiatry Wrong and Psych ER*

Finding the Right Psychiatrist

FINDING THE RIGHT PSYCHIATRIST

A Guide for Discerning Consumers

ROBERT L. TAYLOR, M.D.

Rutgers University Press

New Brunswick, New Jersey, and London

Library of Congress Cataloging–in–Publication Data

Taylor, Robert L., 1942–
Finding the right psychiatrist : a guide for discerning consumers /
Robert L. Taylor, M.D.
    pages cm

Includes bibliographical references and index.
ISBN 978-0-8135-6625-2 (hardcover : alk. paper) — ISBN
978-0-8135-6624-5 (pbk. : alk. paper) — ISBN 978-0-8135-6626-9 (e-book)
Psychiatry—Standards. 2. Psychiatrists—Attitudes. 3. Psychiatrists—
Professional ethics. I. Title.

RC440.8.T38 2014
616.89—dc23   2013037739

A British Cataloging-in-Publication record for this book is available from the
British Library.

Visit our website: http://rutgerspress.rutgers.edu

Manufactured in the United States of America

For Dana Weston

CONTENTS

PREFACE

Before he died, the well-known television personality Mike Wallace spoke candidly about his experiences with severe depression. When asked what he recommended for persons suffering a similar problem, as was his way, he succinctly advised: "Find a good psychiatrist." Commenting on Wallace's straightforward advice, Steven Moffic, a psychiatrist himself, asks: "how does a would-be patient find one?" (Moffic 2012). Choosing the right psychiatrist is complicated, far more complicated than choosing a dermatologist, internist, or plastic surgeon. One main difference is the importance of personality. Your surgeon's personality matters less than his surgical skills. If his hands are good, his personality is less critical. Not so with a psychiatrist. If your psychiatrist's personality gets in the way (and it can), it's a big deal.

A second obstacle to finding a good psychiatrist concerns psychiatry itself. To be sure, this is not the best of times for physicians generally. They struggle with many impediments to good practice including excessive paperwork, interference from managed-care companies, and a relentless demand to see more patients in less time for less pay. Editors at publishing houses describe a deluge of manuscripts from frustrated physicians describing these ordeals. But psychiatrists, while facing similar problems, have an additional challenge. Increasingly, they come under fire for their assumptions about the causes of psychiatric problems and for their views about treatment. Among modern medical specialties, such scrutiny is unique. Although there are always questions about individual care, the merit of medical and surgical specialties themselves seldom is questioned. Among medical disciplines, psychiatry stands alone as the object of such intense scrutiny.

One of my main objectives is to caution you about an unfortunate *narrowing of psychiatric perspective* and to advise you against settling for this. I write about psychiatry from an insider's perspective. I write to champion psychiatry, not to tear it down. While I criticize aspects of traditional psychiatric practice, I do so mainly as a way of describing what it means to be a *complete* psychiatrist. For example, I question the current emphasis on psychiatric diagnoses. Based on long experience, I find them more misleading than helpful. They have a way of reducing patients' unique stories to standard but arbitrary "cases." Although I understand how the official diagnoses listed in the *Diagnostic and Statistical Manual of the American Psychiatric Association* have achieved their prominence (particularly with respect to research and billing), I believe these diagnostic "boxes" promise far more than they deliver. Still, I readily admit that psychiatric diagnoses are here to stay, and I suggest ways they can be used *without* jeopardizing individual care.

You should find a psychiatrist who remains a competent physician, comfortable with matters of mind, brain, and body. Sadly, this broad perspective runs the risk of becoming extinct. In their preoccupation with psychodrugs, many psychiatrists lose interest in psychological and social issues. I'm convinced that a broader-minded psychiatrist—one who combines medical understanding with a proper appreciation of the mind—is best positioned to help his patients. He or she should be expert at recognizing medical conditions that masquerade as psychological problems, including addictions. The frequent intertwining of substance abuse and mental problems makes sensitivity to this toxic combination essential to good psychiatric practice.

Throughout the book you'll find an emphasis on individualized care. Much of what goes on with psychiatric diagnosis and treatment often neglects the individual's particular problems and situations. Despite what psychiatric diagnoses imply, persons with psychiatric conditions—even those who share the same diagnosis—are more different than they are alike. You need a psychiatrist who will treat you as a unique individual.

The question of finding a psychiatrist presumes you *need* a psychiatrist. Not everyone who suffers mood changes, odd behavior, or disturbing thoughts requires psychiatric care. Often these problems prove temporary, resolving as the stresses in a person's life resolve. And even when they persist, they may not indicate a need for psychiatric services. Various therapists, counselors, and personal coaches can provide help with psychological relief as well as guidance on how to minimize stress and change problematic behavior.

But when changes in mood, behavior, and thought become severe enough to disrupt your life, seeing a psychiatrist becomes a reasonable consideration, particularly if medications are required for *immediate* symptom relief. Of the array of mental health professionals, psychiatrists are the only ones with complete medical training who can prescribe psychiatric medications. Additionally, the most severe mental and emotional disruptions frequently need intensive residential or hospital care. Usually, this requires a psychiatric assessment.

Complete medical training also prepares a psychiatrist to recognize psychological masquerades. *Psychological symptoms are not always best explained psychologically.* Sometimes symptoms such as depression and anxiety reflect something other than emotional reactions to life problems. They can be caused by unrecognized medical problems such as thyroid disease, diabetes, and hormonal problems. In fact, when fully evaluated, roughly 10 percent of persons seeking mental health care suffer from underlying medical problems (Taylor 2007). Seeing a psychiatrist who looks for medical problems at the same time he or she helps you sort through various life stressors is a good idea, particularly if you have no previous history of mental and emotional symptoms. Similarly, psychiatric symptoms that come "out of the blue" for no obvious reason deserve a psychiatric evaluation—especially true when these symptoms are associated with medical complaints such as fever or headache.

If you are a person with chronic medical problems, particularly if they require multiple medications, seeing a psychiatrist makes good sense. This is why a psychiatrist is often the best choice for older persons. Also, if you suffer from persistent mental or emotional problems that require psychiatric medications, a psychiatrist is an appropriate choice. The same goes for mental problems complicated by abuse of drugs or alcohol. Having a psychiatrist who is alert to potential medical problems and can prescribe medication for withdrawal and recovery—if needed—will serve you well.

Once you have decided you need a psychiatrist, you may find your choice is limited. In certain areas of the country, they are in short supply. Sometimes you may have to rely on others you trust—physician, minister, family member, or good friend. But in most instances *you* will make a choice. The following chapter provides an overview of some of the obstacles you will face as you search for the right psychiatrist.

ACKNOWLEDGMENTS

Books are easier to write when you have people willing to comment on early versions. I am greatly indebted to Fuller Torrey, Lorrin Koran, Pam Ryan, David Lam, Jerry Lynn, Maxie Weaver, Dana Weston, Paul Minot, and Cynthia Franklin. Their insights made this book far better than it would have been otherwise.

Also, special thanks to my committed agent, Kathleen Davis Niendorff, for guiding the book into publication, to my editor at Rutgers University Press, Dana Dreibelbis, and to my copy editor, Will Hively.

Finally, and far too belatedly, I want to express appreciation to my colleague and friend Maggie Shelby for her support and help with my writing.

Finding the Right Psychiatrist

CHAPTER ONE

What Makes Finding a Psychiatrist So Difficult?

- Look for a complete psychiatrist.

- Select one who is a good therapist as well as a competent prescriber of psychodrugs.

- Avoid the psychiatrist who neglects getting to know who you are.

- Reject the burned-out psychiatrist void of passion for what he or she does.

I've practiced psychiatry more than forty-five years. For the most part, it has been a rewarding journey allowing me to treat patients, design and manage mental health and health programs, lecture, conduct research, explore wellness promotion, and consult on (among other things) the psychological profiles of presidential assassins. Through it all I have found the workings of mind and brain, and the ways human behavior derails and rights itself, endlessly fascinating. Similarly, I have found the relief many patients experience immensely satisfying. But at the end of my career, I am frustrated with psychiatry and psychiatric practice. The things that concern me the most greatly complicate your finding the right psychiatrist.

PSYCHIATRY'S PREDICAMENT

In the not too distant past, psychiatrists made use of insights from psychology, sociology, biology, anthropology, and even philosophy and religion. Of all medical specialists, they seemed best positioned to bridge the worlds of mind and body. Unfortunately, this promise failed to materialize. Psychiatry changed. Many psychiatrists now focus almost exclusively on psychodrugs. This shift would be more understandable if great progress had been made; but, as we will see, despite dramatic neuroscience breakthroughs, few advances have occurred in psychiatric medications. In 2009, Dr. Thomas Insel, director of the National Institute of Mental Health, reluctantly concluded: "Despite high expectations, neither genomics nor imaging has yet impacted the diagnosis or treatment of the 45 million Americans with serious or moderate mental illness each year" (Insel 2009). For decades now psychiatry has awkwardly explained most psychiatric problems as chemical imbalances in need of psychodrugs. This overly narrow interpretation of psychiatric problems has proven detrimental to psychiatrists as well as to their patients.

A recent conversation with a psychiatric colleague illustrates the problem. We had just finished a round of golf. As we walked toward the clubhouse, my friend brushed away my compliment on his approach shot to the eighteenth hole and abruptly announced he was quitting. "Golf?" I asked in disbelief, fully aware of his passion for the sport. "No," he said, "psychiatry." It took a moment for his bombshell to register. From time to time, this man had grumbled about managed health care, but never to the point of actually thinking about giving up psychiatry. We sat down at an outside table for a beer. Clearly he wanted to talk. With an angry, almost hurt edge to his voice, he rambled for several minutes, explaining why after thirty years of psychiatric practice he was done. When he finished, he seemed sad but resolved. After an awkward silence I asked what he planned to do. He didn't know. He was considering taking off a year to decide. The baffled look on my face was enough to keep him talking. "I've had it," he declared with a deep sigh. "I didn't go into psychiatry to see patients for fifteen minutes a pop and write 'scripts.' *Hi, how are you feeling? Any problems? No? Depression better? Great! Here's another Prozac prescription. See you in three months.*" With a disgusted look on his face, he continued: "Patients I've seen for years, I hardly know them. I have no understanding of what's really troubling them. How can I? I spend all my time making diagnoses and prescribing pills." The best I could manage was a sympathetic nod. "It's not good for patients, and it's not good for me," he lamented. I couldn't disagree. While my colleague's decision took me by surprise, the feelings he expressed are not uncommon among psychiatrists. Much of the problem stems from the relentless narrowing of perspective that grips psychiatry.

MIND FOR MOLECULES

Understanding patients—what they hold important, what bothers them, how they trip themselves up, even sabotage their own efforts—no longer serves as a major focus for many psychiatrists. A *New York Times* article titled "Talk Doesn't Pay, So Psychiatry Turns to Drug Therapy" describes how psychiatrists find themselves pressured *not* to do talk therapy with their patients. Doylestown, Pennsylvania, psychiatrist Donald Levin explained the implications: "I had to train myself not to get too interested in their problems" (Harris 2011).

I'm not certain of the instruction psychiatric residents receive these days. How they practice, however, I know well. The relentless demand for recipe-driven assessments, commonly referred to as "med checks," replaces a more comprehensive approach. Concern for the world of mind—the place where, despite brain science advances, we live our lives—becomes an early casualty. After years of clinical experience, one psychiatrist described an "aha" moment when he realized the mistake he had made most of his career (Carlat 2010). A middle-aged man—sleepless and anxious, tortured by a troubled sales job and questionable marriage—came for an initial appointment. After a brief assessment, the psychiatrist reached for his prescription pad. But, for reasons not entirely clear, on this occasion he stopped himself and continued to listen. As it turned out, the moment proved pivotal in this psychiatrist's career as he found himself truly understanding the man's troubled life and sense of failure. In a long-overdue epiphany, the psychiatrist grasped how he had "veered away from psychological curiosity," how "psychiatry had become little more than a repetitive process of labeling patients and finding a drug to match." He saw how this narrow focus had blocked his understanding of patients. "I didn't know what made them tick as people," he admitted. Sadly, a large number of psychiatrists, focused like lasers on chemical imbalance, risk never having this awakening.

Many psychiatrists I've met in recent years complain of feeling burned out. They experience their work as leaving no room for craftsmanship and intellectual stimulation. Already, early in their careers, they lack enthusiasm and passion. Although some understand why—the endless routine of making subjective diagnoses and pushing pills for every problem they encounter—they don't know how to get off the treadmill. Often, in private, they lament their choice of psychiatry as a specialty. They feel that much of what they do (particularly in outpatient settings) resembles fast-food service more than medical specialty practice. Ron Pies, columnist for the *Psychiatric Times* and clinical professor of psychiatry at Tufts University School of Medicine, terms it the "McDonaldization" of psychiatry. (Recently, I came across a job announcement that perfectly captures what they face. The ad called for a psychiatrist who would routinely perform med checks on as many as twenty-eight persons a day!)

Years ago, I filled in as a psychiatrist at a community mental health clinic. As my first patient prepared to leave my office, he shook my hand enthusiastically. "I'm so glad you're my doctor," he said. At the door he turned and finished his thought: "You *look* at me." I smiled without fully understanding. A few days passed before I understood. In this particular clinic psychiatrists spent most of their time with patients writing furiously as they checked off criteria for diagnoses and filled out prescriptions. It was in this context that this patient thanked me for simply looking at him. Unfortunately, this portrayal of many clinical psychiatrists at work is not far off the mark.

In part this nonpersonal approach to psychiatric care relates to the dubious (but prevailing) assumption that psychiatric problems all boil down to the same thing: chemical imbalances. If true, what's the necessity for getting to know patients? Even looking at them? After all, what really matters is ferreting out the specific chemical problem and a pill that will correct it. I urge you to reject any psychiatrist who pays more attention to his or her notes than to you.

Commenting on psychiatry's love affair with psychodrugs, former American Psychiatric Association president Steve Sharfstein, M.D., labeled it the "bio-bio-bio model." He was referring to the domination of biological psychiatry. But his characterization misses the real point if it implies that psychiatrists busy themselves with sophisticated biological explanations of human problems. To the contrary, the razor-thin biological basis of modern psychiatry can be reduced to a single, one-size-fits-all assumption: if it's a psychiatric problem, it's a chemical imbalance. Despite all the marketing verbiage, *no specific chemical imbalance has been established for any psychiatric disorder*. Thus far, revolutionary discoveries in the neurosciences have failed to translate into useful clinical psychiatric insights or tools. In reality, the lionized *biological basis* of psychiatry is more advertising slogan than hard science.

SHAKY FOUNDATION

Throughout its history, the absence of a scientific base has plagued psychiatry. It's why the discipline lurches from one perspective to another. For a while psychiatry saw the world in moral terms. By the nineteenth century, this view was replaced with a primitive biological understanding only to give way again late in the century to a psychological perspective (psychoanalysis). This, in turn, was replaced by brief flirtations with behavioral and then social explanations (community mental health) before the resurrection of a biological view midway through the last century that has persisted to the present. Currently, most psychiatrists emphasize a handful of psychodrugs as the treatment for an expanding list of questionable diagnoses (more about this later), all presumed to reflect various chemical imbalances. Richard Cooper, a professor of medicine at the University of Pennsylvania and an expert on the evolution of medical specialties, explains psychiatry's current preoccupation this way: "Rather than seizing new problems that emerge from technological progress or conceptual growth, it [psychiatry] has expanded its scope of interest by medicalizing what are often referred to as 'problems of living'" (Cooper 2003). In short, unlike other medical specialties that progress by advances in scientific knowledge, psychiatry (in the absence of major advances) tries to create the *appearance of progress* by simply casting its diagnostic net wider and wider.

Given this rickety foundation, psychiatry's future as a medical discipline is by no means a slam dunk. In his book *Psychiatrist on the Road*, Lawrence Climo suggests another possibility when he describes his "untimely retirement." After years as a senior clinical psychiatrist at a New England inner-city mental health clinic, Climo abruptly found himself out of a job. When he asked why, he was told there was nothing personal—just a matter of expense. A nurse could do his work cheaper. End of story (Climo 2009). As the most expensive mental health professionals on the block, psychiatrists are at risk. Tradition and license can hold back the tide only so long against a relentless push for less expensive care. Already, primary care physicians prescribe more psychodrugs than psychiatrists, and nurse practitioners and physician assistants provide far less costly alternatives. Clinical psychologists are coming on strong as they make their play to prescribe psychodrugs. Psychiatrists' routine abandonment of medical skills makes this encroachment easier. The inevitable question will be: why pay for a medical specialist (psychiatrist) if that specialist does not practice medicine?

Increasingly, for many psychiatrists working in public clinics or in private practice, clinical work becomes an onerous endeavor, similar to what my golfing partner described. What was once a multiperspective, highly personalized discipline is reduced largely to, I hate to say it, pill pushing. (Oddly enough, television and film have overlooked this troubling transformation of psychiatry as they persist in portraying psychiatrists as psychotherapists—most often neurotic or bumbling types, full of themselves and unable to maintain professional boundaries. Apparently, the idea of spending one's professional time applying psychiatric diagnoses and handing out pills, day after day, lacks sufficient dramatic potential.)

If you are following this, you will understand what I mean when I refer to "psychiatry's predicament." Many psychiatrists are trapped in unsatisfying practices, attending more to questionable diagnoses and psychodrugs than to understanding their patients. This is the kind of psychiatrist you *don't* want.

DIAGNOSTIC PRETENSIONS

Throughout my career, I have heard predictions of psychiatry's being on the verge of becoming a brain science and of psychiatric conditions being fully revealed as brain diseases. I am still waiting. Despite its aspirations, psychiatry remains a neuroscience pretender. It has built an ever-expanding array of diagnostic categories without any causative understanding. In real life, precisely described "disorders," more often than not, turn out to be various blends of troubled emotions, thoughts, and behaviors. Clear diagnostic distinctions occur only in the pages of the *DSM* (*Diagnostic and Statistical Manual*). You want a psychiatrist who resists assigning you to a diagnostic box and insisting all your problems fit that label.

Ironically, despite the emphasis on official psychiatric diagnoses, for the most part, when it comes to prescribing psychodrugs, it's not diagnoses but rather *symptoms* that psychiatrists target. There is an obvious reason for this. Whether we are talking about schizophrenia, bipolar disorder, major depression, borderline personality, ADHD, or obsessive-compulsive disorder, the precise cause remains unknown. To the degree they work, psychodrugs minimize or alleviate various *symptoms*—depression, mania, anxiety, obsessions, compulsions, hallucinations, delusions—experienced by patients with different diagnoses. Upon hearing my critique of psychiatric diagnoses, one of my colleagues insisted I was being unfair. After all, he argued, most medical diseases are not fully understood, and the actions of many general medications remain unknown. Often, they—like psychodrugs—provide only symptomatic relief. So, the difference between psychiatry and medicine, he insisted, is simply a matter of degree. He makes a good point, but the degree of difference is *huge*. In contrast to many medical and neurological conditions, there are *no* established biological causes for *any* psychiatric disorder. You may have heard "brain abnormalities" cited as causes. What passes for a brain abnormality invariably turns out to be statistical differences found in only a small percentage of patients. Lest you think I am a hopeless Luddite, I do not rule out a future where biological understanding sheds greater light on mental and emotional problems and where biological treatments are more efficacious. But regardless of what you have heard, that future is not now, and no one knows how long it will be before it arrives. Walk away from any psychiatrist who tells you otherwise.

Medical students follow closely the future prospects for various medical specialties. When they decide to go into pediatrics or hematology or family medicine, in part it's because they believe the discipline has a bright future. Over the past forty years, the percentage of medical students choosing psychiatry has dropped dramatically, now less than a quarter of what it was in the late 1960s. Increasingly, those selecting psychiatry are foreign medical graduates. Psychiatry's troubles likely play an important part in this declining interest in the discipline. In his 1974 book *The Death of Psychiatry*, Fuller Torrey argued that since most psychiatric patients suffer from problems in living rather than true medical conditions, psychiatry was in deep trouble. Such problems, he contended, would be better addressed with psychotherapy than with pills or medical procedures. In the absence of any compelling evidence that psychiatrists were superior psychotherapists, he predicted an untimely death for psychiatry (Torrey 1974). Technically, Torrey was wrong, at least up to now. Psychiatry remains alive, though some would say not by much. At the very least, it's fair to say, the discipline is having a rough time.

OVERSELLING PSYCHODRUGS

For more than a dozen years, I have practiced psychiatry in a variety of treatment settings—community mental health clinics, psychiatric hospitals, emergency mental health services, jails, and prisons. Without exception, these programs have emphasized psychodrugs to the relative exclusion of other treatments. Several months ago, I had dinner with friends—all well educated and sophisticated about things psychological. In the course of conversation my brief mention of the sad state of psychodrugs was met with disbelieving looks. What about all those television ads, they asked, all the new psychiatric drugs? I had a hard time convincing them otherwise. I suspect, as you read this, you may have a similar reaction. So I'll say it more emphatically: *there has been no improvement in psychodrug efficacy over the past fifty years.* The side effects have changed, but effectiveness remains the same. In our over-reliance on psychodrugs, psychiatrists tie ourselves to a dormant treatment riddled with adverse effects and often no more effective than placebos. To complicate matters, with respect to various classes of psychodrugs—antidepressants, antipsychotics, anxiety meds, and mood stabilizers—no solid basis exists for selecting one drug over another for any particular patient. Apart from a consideration of side effects, and a patient's previous psychodrug history (or the experience of a closely related relative), choice of psychiatric medication remains more guessing game than careful determination.

Despite these difficulties, in a later chapter I describe what I consider the invaluable role psychodrugs sometimes play, and I discuss instances of severe mental and emotional problems for which there are no reasonable alternatives. But for the moment, this is the take-home message: though important tools, psychodrugs are not all they are cracked up to be, and they tend to be overused.

CHAMPIONS OF THE STATUS QUO

So, how did psychiatry come to this? How did a discipline that forty years ago attracted 10–15 percent of all medical graduates lose its way? Much of the credit goes to four players: pharmaceutical companies, psychiatric academia, organized psychiatry, and managed care. Collectively and often in lockstep they have fashioned present-day psychiatry and, as far as I can tell, seem reasonably content with the outcome. It is unlikely any of these players will instigate or encourage major changes.

Pharmaceutical companies specializing in psychiatric medications have been thrilled with the way psychiatry has evolved, since their major commitment is to stockholders for whom they have done exceedingly well by exuberantly promoting the myth of chemical imbalance and the corrective benefits of psychodrugs. With millions at stake, predictably, they will use their influence to keep things as they are.

By and large psychodrugs are the major focus of Psychiatry Department chairmen. Through research and education grants, academic psychiatry has close ties to pharmaceutical companies. Most academic psychiatry careers today are built on psychodrugs, and psychopharmacology remains the undisputed king of the psychiatric training curriculum. Many Psychiatry Department chairmen retain cozy relationships with psychopharma companies, thus ensuring that an ongoing cloud of vested interest hangs over psychiatric training institutions. Even so, there's little reason to think a move away from psychodrugs by department chairmen is imminent.

A third player certain to resist psychiatric change is the American Psychiatric Association (APA)—the national trade organization of psychiatrists. Again, the resistance comes down to money. A 2006 report of financial ties of psychiatrist panel members working on the newest APA-sponsored diagnostic manual (*DSM-IV*) turned up some disturbing facts: "Of the 170 DSM panel members, 95 (56%) had one or more financial associations with companies in the pharmaceutical industry. One hundred per cent of the members of the panels on 'Mood

Disorders' and 'Schizophrenia and Other Psychotic Disorders' had financial ties. . . . The leading categories of financial interest held by panel members were research funding (42%), consultancies (22%), and speakers bureau (16%)" (Cosgrove et al. 2006). Given the expense of numerous committees that require paid travel and accommodations for meetings, the APA, with its dwindling membership, depends critically on continued psychodrug company support. Based on 2008 figures, a *New York Times* investigation showed roughly 30 percent of the APA's annual budget coming from the drug industry (Carey and Gardiner 2008). Even though recent *unofficial* reports from APA staff suggest that the organization has responded to critics by reducing the organization's dependence on psychopharma financial support, it is unlikely the APA will be a major change agent in shifting the focus of psychiatry away from psychodrugs.

In the early 1970s, a group of optimistic, young psychiatrists set out to give redirection to the APA. The group took advantage of a long-forgotten bylaw allowing for an alternate slate of officers by petition. For years only a single, unopposed slate of officers had been nominated. It was a closed club. If you got to be treasurer, you could be sure that a few years later you would ascend to the presidency. The Committee of Concerned Psychiatrists put forward an alternative list of candidates chosen for their progressive views and, two years later, ran the table. Alternative candidates won all the national positions. But what initially passed as a heady moment of political triumph turned, within a few years, into dismay as these newly elected officers became co-opted by special interests. The APA doesn't lead so much as it follows the money; and, for years, this strategy has led straight to the doors of various psychodrug companies. Some habits are hard to break.

Finally, there is managed care. These health-care gatekeepers are more than content to have psychiatric problems reduced to chemical imbalances. Pills are much simpler (and less costly) than more subjective psychotherapies. Managed-care companies have been remarkably effective at arbitrarily barring psychiatrists from practicing psychotherapy, despite evidence that a combined approach is more cost effective (Dewan 1999).

PSYCHIATRY AT THE CROSSROADS

So serious is psychiatry's predicament, one close observer advises a major redo of the profession. In his book *Unhinged*, psychiatrist Daniel Carlat declares psychiatry a failed discipline (2010). He recommends psychiatrists re-engineer themselves into super psychologists. I read Dr. Carlat's book with great interest. He does a good job describing psychiatry's plight, but his suggested remedy I can't buy. To the contrary I believe psychiatry's most promising future lies ahead *if* it can make itself a deserving *discipline* by establishing itself as a *mindful* medical specialty.

Patients need a medical discipline that embraces mind and body, and the field of medicine would be enhanced by a true mind-body specialty. This role is psychiatry's for the asking, but only if it remakes itself. As it stands, psychiatry hangs on as a *pretender* medical discipline. No other branch of medicine has shown so little substantive progress. A psychiatrist could have dropped out of the profession in the 1970s, joined the Peace Corps, served for forty years, and then resurfaced and taken up practice again with minimal extra training. Unless there are major changes, psychiatry's future appears bleak. Medical students will continue to pass it by. Psychiatrists risk remaining stuck in a one-dimensional view of human problems, dependent on a single tool—psychodrugs—doing what other professionals can do equally well until eventually they find themselves priced out of the market.

This is all by way of background as you prepare yourself to look for the right psychiatrist. You can't just assume that because a psychiatrist's credentials are all in order he or she is right for you. Many "certified" psychiatrists will not deviate from the mantra of chemical imbalance. Fortunately, there are others who remain more flexible and imaginative in how they practice. This is the kind of psychiatrist you should search out. To be sure, you want him or her to be technically competent, but you also want a psychiatrist who listens and gets to know you and your special story and who has a tool kit with more than one tool in it.

For good reason, standard psychiatric practice has come under substantial attack. You can't afford to leave your choice of a psychiatrist to the Yellow Pages (Angell 2011b; Oldham, Carlat, et al. 2011). In this introductory chapter, I've provided an overview of major fracture lines in psychiatry. Because of the basic assumptions they make, many psychiatrists will not be right for you. One of your most important considerations should be how a psychiatrist approaches psychiatric diagnosis, a topic I discuss in the following chapter.

CHAPTER TWO

Psychiatric Diagnosis

The Problem with Boxes

- Avoid the psychiatrist who thinks your diagnosis more important than you.

- Understand psychiatric diagnoses for what they are: arbitrary categories.

- Choose a psychiatrist who understands that psychiatric diagnoses can be more misleading than helpful.

- Reject being treated as a diagnosed "case."

There's a certain magic attached to naming things.

A name implies understanding. Confronted with a puzzling world of troubled behaviors, thoughts, and emotions, psychiatry carves out discrete psychiatric disorders. After all, this is what medicine does. Unfortunately, what works for medicine doesn't work for psychiatry.

Psychiatric diagnosis has a long history of notable detractors. Decades ago, the respected Canadian psychiatrist Heinz

Lehman labeled it "a superficial, unconvincing, and . . . useless procedure." Robert Litman, UCLA professor of psychiatry and creator of the nation's first suicide prevention center, went even further, referring to psychiatric diagnosis as "pseudo-science"; and, with characteristic bluntness, Karl Menninger dismissed it as "verbal Mickey Mouse." Despite these dismal appraisals, psychiatric diagnoses persist and now dominate mental health care. If you go to a psychiatrist, chances are you will be given one. That's why you need to understand them for what they are.

HOW AND WHY PSYCHIATRIC DIAGNOSES GREW

Psychiatric diagnoses evolved relatively late. Oddly enough, the first semiofficial listing appeared in the 1840 United States census as a single category: idiocy/insanity. By 1880, there were 7 categories: mania, melancholia, monomania, paresis, dementia, dipsomania, and epilepsy. It would be forty more years before psychiatry came up with its own list of 22 diagnoses—most of them organic mental disorders—in what was titled the *Statistical Manual for the Use of Institutions for the Insane* (modeled after an old military manual). From this point forward the list of psychiatric disorders expanded and morphed its way through various versions until it achieved official status in 1952 as *DSM-I*, the first *Diagnostic and Statistical Manual of the American Psychiatric Association*. This 130-page manual included 106 diagnoses. By 1980 the number had grown to 265 in *DSM-III*. Fourteen years later 365 diagnoses were listed in the 886-page *DSM-IV* (Blashfield 1998).

You might interpret this relentless growth of official disorders as a sign of notable progress: psychiatry at work unearthing previously unknown psychiatric conditions. Sadly, this is not the case. Unlike in medicine, where most diagnoses have identifiable causes backed by objective tests, psychiatric diagnoses are subjective characterizations, based solely on history and symptoms *without known causes or objective confirmatory evidence.*

Consider the following example. As gay/lesbian issues and rights surfaced in the 1970s, the American Psychiatric Association was pressured to remove "homosexuality" from its list of psychiatric disorders. Finally, simply on the basis of a *vote* of the membership, the diagnosis was expunged. In an instant, roughly 1.5 million gay and lesbian persons became "undiagnosed," deemed no longer to suffer from a psychiatric disorder. (Not that they ever did. I mention the incident only to emphasize the subjective nature of psychiatric diagnoses.)

But if psychiatric diagnoses have no objective confirmation, what drives their growth? Some observers claim that much of it relates to the relentless "medicalization" of variations of normal behavior. And given some of the *DSM* listings, the claim would seem to have some merit. Consider the following *DSM* disorders: rumination (307.53), (mis)conduct (312.89), oppositional defiant (313.81), insomnia (780.52), hoarding (300.3), and dependent personality (301.6). If these variants qualify as official diagnoses, the potential for new *DSM* listings appears unlimited.

SUBJECTIVE LABELS

Over a century ago, the psychiatric pioneer Emil Kraepelin concluded in frustration: "As long as we are unable clinically to group illnesses on the basis of cause and to separate dissimilar causes, our views about etiology will necessarily remain unclear and contradictory" (Shorter 2009). In this regard, nothing has changed since Kraepelin. *DSM* diagnoses remain subjective descriptions, constructed by committees, absent definitive biological evidence such as laboratory tests, tissue biopsies, imaging results, or genetic typing. I don't think most patients understand this limitation. In fact, many mental health professionals misconstrue psychiatric disorders as discrete illnesses.

The American Psychiatric Association (the official overseer of psychiatric diagnosis) perpetuates this confusion in its introductory comments on the *DSM*: "The naming of categories is the traditional method of organizing and transmitting information . . . used in all systems of medical diagnosis" (*DSM-IV-TR* 2000). True, but for the most part medical diagnoses are based on objective findings. In contrast, psychiatric disorders arise out of committee discussion and are powered by special interests. This inherent subjectivity leads to a number of predictable problems.

For example, psychiatric diagnoses commonly change.

Anyone who reviews psychiatric records quickly becomes familiar with shifting diagnoses. A person presents with *"mood swings."* For a time he or she is labeled *cyclothymic personality*, only to have the diagnosis replaced eventually with *bipolar disorder I* and later still with *bipolar disorder II*. And, with another slight shift in symptoms, the diagnosis may change yet again to *psychotic disorder, unspecified* or *schizoaffective disorder*.

Subjectivity also contributes to the high rate of multiple psychiatric diagnoses (known as comorbidity). Although understandable as an infrequent occurrence, when almost *half* of psychiatric patients have multiple diagnoses, the validity of the diagnoses becomes questionable.

In truth, most psychiatric problems are a blend of symptoms and disabilities that cut across various diagnoses. In their complexity and uniqueness, they defy relegation to discrete diagnostic boxes, a fact guaranteed to perplex committees charged with coming up with official psychiatric diagnoses. The outcome is inevitable: committee groupthink airbrushes away the real-world blurring of diagnostic boundaries in favor of precise *DSM* categories (with their exact numerical codes).

The vagaries of *DSM* diagnoses are illustrated in major league baseball's experience with ADHD (attention deficit/hyperactivity disorder). In 2006 28 major league players had a diagnosis of ADHD. By 2011 the number had increased to 105. One NIMH psychiatrist pointed out that major league baseball players were twice as likely to have ADHD as members of the general population (fourteen- to forty-four-year-olds). There's no way to prove it, but the most likely explanation for this finding lies in the subjectivity of the diagnosis, which, in this case, opens the door to "legitimate" use of performance-enhancing stimulants. If you want a diagnosis of ADHD, likely you can get it, in part, because this diagnosis—like other *DSM* diagnoses—remains imprecisely applied without confirmatory biological markers (Moore and Corbett 2012). This has caused colleges to have to clamp down on students who claim they have ADHD as a means of securing "uppers." A recent *New York Times* report describes unusual actions by the Student Health Office at Fresno State University (California). Before they can receive a prescription for a stimulant medication, students with "ADHD" must now submit to drug testing, agree to see a mental health professional monthly, and promise not to share pills (Schwarz 2013).

PUFFING UP THE *DSM*

In 1980 *DSM-III* adopted a major change, deemed at the time a significant diagnostic advance—so much so that it was carried over to the next version, *DSM-IV*. In this new "multiaxial" psychiatric diagnostic scheme, a single diagnosis was no longer sufficient; instead, five separate assessments were required: Axis I—the primary clinical disorder(s); Axis II—personality disorders and mental retardation (developmental disabilities); Axis III— general medical conditions; Axis IV—psychosocial and environmental stressors; and Axis V—global assessment of functioning (GAF). Unfortunately, rather than being a true advance in psychiatric diagnosis, this multiaxial format provided cover for *DSM*'s uninspired perpetuation of subjective, artificial categories.

In actual practice, this "advanced" diagnostic system worked like this. A patient's "presenting" problem (major depressive disorder, bipolar disorder, generalized anxiety disorder) was listed as the Axis I diagnosis. Axis II, supposedly an in-depth appraisal of personality, typically consisted of little more than throwaway comments such as "none," "deferred," or "by history." Over the years, "Axis II" evolved into a pejorative tag applied to troublesome patients. An example recently came to light in a report of U.S. soldiers being diagnosed with "personality disorders" as a way of discharging them for troublesome ("maladaptive") behavior. Headlines described a woman captain expelled from the service as a "personality disorder" in response to orders from higher-ups. Since 2001, at least thirty-one thousand service members have been discharged from the military for vaguely defined "personality disorders" (Dao 2012).

Axis III was the place for medical diagnoses. Here, some psychiatrists provided a full list of all complicating major medical problems; others left it blank, partly completed, or with notations such as "none known" or "deferred." The thoroughness varied considerably.

Axis IV called for an appraisal of psychosocial factors. While such factors often play an important role in patients' stories, the usual entries for this axis were throw-away comments such as "stressed" or "problem relationship." Listing something seemed far more important than thoroughness.

As for Axis V, it was completely bogus.

The other name for Axis V was GAF, global assessment of functioning scale, supposedly a measurement of multiple factors—cognition, functioning, psychotic thought, suicidality—all reduced to a single number between 0 and 100. In actuality, with no objective basis for assigning numbers, GAF was clinically worthless. Only insurers and regulators paid much attention. Payment—not clinical considerations—was its main determinant. Typically, the GAF score turned out to be whatever was necessary for a service to be billed.

In short, the multiaxial *DSM* diagnostic format—while implying a major advance in psychiatric diagnosis—was little more than puffed-up clutter. Luckily, after many years, it has now been officially rejected in *DSM-5*.

DSM-5: UNFULFILLED PROMISE

In December 2012 the American Psychiatric Association approved a fifth edition of the *DSM*, which began arriving in stores May 2013 (American Psychiatric Association 2013). Expectations that this new version of *DSM* would put psychiatric diagnosis on a more solid footing quickly faded when it became obvious that no breakthroughs were forthcoming. The problems of earlier versions remain in *DSM-5*. An array of symptoms are made to appear as objectively based diagnoses. Specific disorders materialize from what most often are overlapping categories. Consequently, the diagnoses continue to mislead more than help by reducing individual stories and situations to sterile and coded but artificial "cases."

At its core, *DSM-5* remains unchanged from *DSM-IV*.

A few disorders are deleted, a few added. Overall, the number remains about the same. Gone is the "grief exemption" that precluded diagnosing persons with major depression within two weeks of losing a loved one. Of course, this means more diagnoses in the future. Gambling now qualifies as a *non-substance addiction*. (Excessive shopping, too much sex, Internet and video preoccupation will have to wait another time; the reasoning for this distinction remains unclear.) The officializing of *binge-eating disorder* (overeating at least once a week for three months) and *somatic symptom disorder* (a six-month preoccupation with health concerns) provides more evidence for the claim that *DSM* grows by codifying variations of normal behavior. A similar concern has been expressed about the newly minted *disruptive mood dysregulation disorder*. Looking like a proxy for temper tantrums, this new diagnosis increases the chances of yet another false spike in child psychiatric diagnoses.

The most hotly debated *DSM-5* proposal was *"pre-psychotic disorder."* This would have provided an official diagnosis for behavior suggestive of *pending* psychosis. Ultimately, the concept proved unworkable, the prediction too complicated. One researcher claimed its inclusion would produce 70–75 percent false diagnoses of persons who met the criteria but would never develop psychosis (Yung et al. 2007). Robert Spitzer, Columbia University professor of psychiatry and chief architect of *DSM-III*, weighed in on the matter. "There will be adolescents who are a little odd and have funny ideas, and this will label them as pre-psychotic" (AOL News 2010). When the dust settled, "pre-psychotic" failed to qualify for *DSM-5*.

Although largely unheralded, the prize for most significant change in *DSM-5* probably goes to the elimination of the vaunted five-axis format. Thirty-three years after its inception, this cumbersome pretense of advanced psychiatric diagnosis was finally retracted, a welcomed change, but hardly a major advance.

After fifteen hundred experts deliberated for many years, *DSM-5*, appearing as much-ado-about-nothing, sparked a surprisingly energized media response, mostly critical.

> "How Psychiatry Went Crazy"
> (Carol Tavris, *Wall Street Journal*, May 17, 2013)
>
> "Psychiatry's Guide Is Out of Touch with Science, Experts Say"
> (Pam Belluck and Benedict Carey, *New York Times*, May 6, 2013)
>
> "A Manual Run Amok: It's Time for Psychiatry to Drop Its Field Guide and Try to Learn About Mental Ills"
> (Paul McHugh, *Wall Street Journal*, May 18/19, 2013)
>
> "Shortcomings of a Psychiatric Bible"
> (Editorial Board, *New York Times*, May 11, 2013)
>
> "Shrink Wrapping: A Single Book Has Come to Dominate Psychiatry"
> (*Economist*, May 18, 2013)

This intense scrutiny of *DSM-5* on the eve of its publication highlighted the unsatisfactory nature of *DSM* thinking itself. Dr. McHugh, a Distinguished Professor of Psychiatry at Johns Hopkins, summed it up this way: "*DSM-5* is a missed opportunity to advance the discipline, instruct the public and encourage financial support for needed psychiatric services. Its editors seem willing to waste another decade before dispersing the mysteries of psychiatry and bringing practitioners and patients together in understanding what they are doing and why" (McHugh 2013).

Even the director of the National Institute of Mental Health, Dr. Thomas R. Insel, blasted *DSM-5*, insisting it failed to "reflect the complexity of many disorders" and cautioning against its use in psychiatric research (Belluck and Carey 2013).

Establishing the reliability of psychiatric diagnoses was one of the major goals of *DSM-5* developers, but this was not to be. In *The Book of Woe*, Gary Greenberg provides an insider account of how field trials aimed at establishing *DSM-5* reliability collapsed when only 195 of 5,000 clinicians followed through with training. Of those who finished, only 70 enrolled *any* patients in clinical trials. To further complicate matters, two months before trials were scheduled to finish, only a few had even gotten under way (Greenberg 2013). In the end, despite the APA's initial goal of 10,000 field trial patients, only 150 actually participated.

The challenge of establishing clinical reliability of psychiatric diagnoses has gone unmet for quite a while. In 1973 a widely discussed report titled *On Being Sane in Insane Places* by Stanford professor David Rosenhan raised serious questions about psychiatric diagnoses (Rosenhan 1973). As part of Rosenhan's study, eight pseudopatients—persons without psychiatric disorders, pretending otherwise—got themselves admitted to twelve different psychiatric hospitals by claiming they heard strange sounds. Once admitted, they acted normal and denied any further symptoms. Even so, all were labeled "psychotic." On average they remained hospitalized nineteen days, and on leaving, all but one were diagnosed *schizophrenia in remission*. In understated fashion, Rosenhan concluded that psychiatric diagnoses appeared imprecise and heavily influenced by the settings in which they were used. These findings sparked a heated debate. Were psychiatric diagnoses to be trusted? A major study was undertaken for clarification. The results proved even more disturbing. The well-respected psychiatric researchers concluded: "There are no diagnostic categories for which reliability is uniformly high. . . . The level of reliability is no better than fair for psychosis and schizophrenia and is poor for the remaining categories" (Spitzer and Fleiss 1974).

The shadow over *DSM* persists in its fifth version: its diagnoses remain unreliable. Even so, given its captive audience, the manual likely will remain the gold standard of mental health assessment and will have huge sales. (Reportedly, *DSM-IV* has sold over a million copies!) In a nutshell, this means that even for well-established psychiatric diagnoses—schizophrenia, bipolar disorder, schizoaffective disorder—there's a good chance that any two psychiatrists will disagree.

For consumers, the message is clear: don't take psychiatric diagnoses too seriously. Make certain you choose a psychiatrist who does likewise. If this is a problem for the psychiatrist, find another. Understanding a person in the context of his or her individual story—personality, situation, symptoms, and history—remains far more valuable than an official psychiatric diagnosis. Over my career I have become increasingly disenchanted with these contrived labels and now believe that *DSM* diagnoses are more misleading than helpful. Let me explain.

LABELING GONE WILD

In their book *Sway*, Ori and Rom Brafman describe the "bipolar epidemic." This explosion of bipolar diagnoses started with a seemingly minor change in *DSM-III*. Persons with less severe manic symptoms now qualified for the diagnosis, and previous hospitalization was no longer required. The consequences were unanticipated. Soon, far more persons were being diagnosed "bipolar." Quick to see the profit implications, psychodrug companies jumped onto the bandwagon and aggressively promoted this new bipolar lite. They subsidized new journals featuring bipolar disorder, organized bipolar support groups, and released a blitz of promotional television ads—all of which made for a huge snowball effect. "The more bipolar disorder was placed in the spotlight, the more clinicians were exposed to it, the higher the diagnosis rate climbed, which in turn led to further diagnosing" (Brafman and Brafman 2008).

Bipolar fever quickly spread to child psychiatry.

In 1994, 25 out of every 100,000 American children were diagnosed bipolar. By 2003 the number had grown fortyfold. At the height of the "epidemic," bipolar diagnoses were being given to two- and three-year-olds! The first hint that these might be false diagnoses was the failure of other psychiatric diagnoses to show an increase. In addition, a questionable disparity emerged. Ordinarily, patients with bona fide bipolar disorder are at greater risk for suicide; but, during this "manufactured" explosion of bipolar diagnoses, suicides actually dropped by 23 percent. Together these findings strongly suggested that many of the new bipolar diagnoses were invalid.

This epidemic of pseudo bipolar diagnoses serves as a glaring example of the wayward potential of *DSM* diagnoses. Once "officialized," you can bet on it—a psychiatric diagnosis will be applied, even when it's not merited. ("If you build it, they will come.") In the case of the bipolar epidemic, unnecessary treatment with antipsychotic drugs became a major liability. This is why some commentators now question *DSM-5*'s new category— *disruptive mood dysregulation disorder*. The diagnosis supposedly describes children over the age of six with frequent tantrums, angry outbursts, and irritability. But what's to keep it from being applied to children who simply do things and say things that grown-ups don't approve of or don't have the time and energy to deal with? Children who by temperament are moody or stubborn may well find themselves targets of this newly minted *DSM* category (Carey 2010b).

Appearing on the Public Broadcast System *NewsHour* on February 10, 2010, chairman of the earlier *DSM-IV* task force Allen Frances claimed that past changes in *DSM-IV* have caused three false spikes in psychiatric diagnoses. In addition to *childhood bipolar disorder*, he named *autism* and *attention deficit disorder*. Such spikes have far-reaching implications, starting with the liability of having to live with a false psychiatric diagnosis. Add to this the risks associated with unnecessary treatment. For example, most children and adolescents diagnosed with ADHD take prescribed stimulant medications for extended periods. What is the long-term effect? After all, these medications resemble cocaine and methamphetamine. The answer is: we really don't know. New guidelines in *DSM-5* increase the likelihood of overdiagnosing ADHD. With an increase in maximum age of onset (from seven to twelve years) and with objective evidence of impairment no longer required, diagnoses are sure to escalate (Frances 2010).

If you are following me, you will understand when I say: with respect to psychiatric diagnoses, *buyer beware*. They are not what they seem. Regardless of which psychiatrist you choose, accept *no* psychiatric diagnosis at face value. Expect your psychiatrist to personalize his assessment (and treatment as well) beyond any official *DSM* diagnosis.

FURTHER DOWNSIDE

In his intriguing book *Plato Not Prozac!* Lou Marinoff likens *DSM* diagnosis to practices in the Middle Ages. When asked why opium put people to sleep, healers of the day said it had *dormative properties* (coming from the Latin word *dormier*, to sleep). Essentially, they were asserting (in "technical language," of course) that opium put people to sleep because it put them to sleep (Marinoff 1999). Much of the *DSM* suffers from similar circular reasoning. The anxious patient becomes an "anxiety disorder"; depressed, a "depressive disorder"; oppositional, an "oppositional defiant disorder"; and badly behaving, a "conduct disorder." Like its medieval precursor, *DSM* labeling often becomes little more than restating your complaint in official diagnostic terms. Given a society that still attaches considerable stigma to "mental illness," this form of diagnosis-for-the-sake-of-diagnosis seems particularly egregious.

In a book titled *Doing Psychiatry Wrong: A Critical and Prescriptive Look at a Faltering Profession*, René Muller criticizes the *DSM* for ignoring the personal meaning of symptoms. Even for those persons who benefit from psychodrugs, there remains the important task of making sense of disturbing symptoms. Unfortunately, too often, such help fails to materialize from psychiatrists (Muller 2008). Psychiatric evaluation should go beyond diagnosis. You want a psychiatrist who in addition to treating your symptoms helps you understand them. Even if your symptoms persist, you need a psychiatrist who will explore with you how to live with them, integrate them into your life, and make them less disruptive.

One of the unappreciated risks of *DSM* diagnoses stems from how they sometimes obscure other problems. Consider ADHD again. Unfortunately, many children receive this diagnosis in error. Restless kids who can't concentrate and who act impulsively don't all suffer from this condition. Like other psychiatric disorders, ADHD is not the discrete "illness" it's made out to be; rather, it's a syndrome: a collection of symptoms that arise from various causes. One leader in the field, Dr. Joel Nigg, says it this way: "ADHD represents not a single disease entity

but a heterogeneous group of patients who require differenti-
ated analysis, assessment, and treatment" (Nigg 2009).

Sometimes attention/hyperactivity symptoms result from
specific learning deficits related to reading, writing, spelling,
and math—deficits that can be confirmed only with special neu-
ropsychological testing. Similarly, ADHD symptoms can be the
expression of a variety of medical masquerades, including low
blood sugar, overactive thyroid, high levels of lead or mercury,
iron deficiency, and hearing deficits. Adverse side effects from
medications, addiction, and faulty vision can all mimic ADHD.

A Sunday *New York Times* front-page article titled "Drowned
in a Stream of Prescriptions" detailed the tragic life of a college
graduate treated with Adderall (a stimulant) for ADHD. Somewhere along the way the student became addicted and developed
a stimulant-induced psychosis. Even so, he continued to secure a
supply of medication from multiple doctors for treatment of his
"ADHD." Eventually his father discovered him dead in the closet
of his apartment, having hanged himself (Schwarz 2013).

The standard treatment for ADHD when applied to "look-
alike" conditions may prevent the use of more effective treatments. Sometimes an overactive, inattentive child best profits
from special training in attention, listening, and thinking before
acting or in other nonmedication interventions (such as computer
simulations and monitored video games) aimed at enhancing
self-control and concentration. In a *New York Times* op-ed piece
titled "Ritalin Gone Wrong," University of Minnesota psychology professor emeritus Alan Sroufe explains why these interventions don't happen as often as they should. "Policy makers are so
convinced that children with attention deficits have an organic
disease that they have all but called off the search for a comprehensive understanding " (Sroufe 2012). He goes on to describe

how research scientists, aware of this bias, submit grant requests targeted mainly at the biochemistry of ADHD.

Even with major mental disorders such as schizophrenia—now considered by many a brain disease—*DSM* diagnosis can mislead. All psychiatric conditions—including schizophrenia and bipolar disorder—are more spectrum in nature than they are distinct categories. This means that patients with identical diagnoses are more different than similar. One Swiss study investigated 289 patients (age sixty-five or older) with schizophrenia. Roughly half had an initial, acute psychotic episode; the other half, a slow, "insidious" onset. Later on, again, roughly half suffered psychotic episodes followed by much calmer periods in contrast to the other half, who were continuously psychotic. Similarly, the long-term outcome split down the middle. Half of the patients had moderate to severe disability while the other half had only mild disability and, in 25percent of cases, fully recovered (Ciompi 1980). Here we have persons with life-long disabling symptoms and persons who fully recover or at least recover enough to attend college, marry, have children, and hold jobs lumped together in the same diagnostic box—*schizophrenia*. Too often mental health clinics (and many psychiatrists) assume *all* persons with "schizophrenia" have a lifelong debilitating illness that necessitates antipsychotic medication on a continuous basis. For a significant number of persons, this characterization grossly misleads. Such is the distorting power of *DSM* diagnoses.

Compare prevailing beliefs with what pioneering psychiatric researcher Dr. Courtney Harding says about schizophrenia: (1) Contrary to the idea "once a schizophrenic, always a schizophrenic," persons with "schizophrenia" have better than an even chance of greatly improving or recovering. (2) Lumping together all persons with this diagnosis ignores the fact that they are more different than alike. "Attention to individual differences, life histories, and developmental steps, will encourage patients to perceive themselves, *not* as 'schizophrenics,' but rather as people, who happen to have schizophrenia." (3) Rehabilitation efforts are *not* a waste of time, and they need not be delayed until a person is completely stabilized. (4) Psychotherapy is as applicable to the lives of people with schizophrenia as anyone else. Perhaps more so. Problems in living are problems in living. We all have them. (5) Contrary to psychiatric tradition, only a "small percentage" of these persons need medication indefinitely. (6) Persons with schizophrenia "can and do perform at every level of work." (7) Despite a lingering myth, "No evidence exists that a family's psychosocial climate, communication patterns, or parenting practices are primary causes of schizophrenia." To the contrary, families and significant others, if mobilized, can provide invaluable social support, practical help, and encouragement (Harding and Zahniser 1994).

In this age of social media, "family" often includes more than relatives. Take, for example, the Hearing Voices Network (started by Dutch psychiatrist Marius Romme and his colleague Dr. Sandra Escher)—an international organization of patients and nonpatients who share a common experience: hearing voices. One of the organization's core assumptions is that hearing voices by itself is not a sign of mental illness, a challenging concept for *DSM*.

In a 1998 *American Journal of Psychiatry* editorial article, Gary Tucker said this about *DSM* diagnosis: "we have lost the patient and his or her story with this process. . . . the diagnosis, not the patient, often gets treated. . . . surprisingly, the study of psychopathology is almost nonexistent . . . and . . . the strict focus on diagnosis has made psychiatry boring" (Tucker 1998). Tucker borrowed a page from Hippocrates, who centuries ago admonished general physicians to focus on the person. "It's more important to know what sort of person has a disease," he insisted, "than to know what sort of disease a person has." It's an important admonition for all physicians, but particularly for psychiatrists. Overlooked too often is how *DSM* diagnoses serve as obstacles to understanding individual patients.

The philosopher Martin Buber distinguished two kinds of human relationship (Buber 1958). I-Thou relationships he characterized as personal and respectful, whereas I-It relationships are instrumental and nonpersonal. Psychiatric diagnoses encourage I-It doctor-patient relationships. Patients run the risk of becoming diagnosed "cases" rather than unique persons with their own stories and situations. Good for billing and research efforts, psychiatric diagnoses prove much less beneficial as clinical guides.

Too often diagnoses transform individuals into standard cases. I'll never forget a patient who reminded me of this long after I thought I fully understood. I don't recall my exact words, but they were something along the lines of his needing to accept being "bipolar." With a quizzical look, the young man stared at me for several beats and then said: "But I'm not bipolar. That's just my diagnosis." Touché!

Irv Yalom, one of my psychiatry professors at Stanford and author of several classic textbooks on psychotherapy, said it this way: "A diagnosis limits vision; it diminishes ability to relate to the other person. Once we make a diagnosis, we tend to selectively inattend to aspects of the patient that do not fit into that particular diagnosis, and correspondingly over attend to subtle features that appear to confirm an initial diagnosis." He went on to speculate: "Undoubtedly, the time will come when the

DSM-IV Chinese restaurant menu format will appear ludicrous to mental health professionals" (Yalom 2002). Given the lock *DSM* has on the field, this may be an overly optimistic prediction.

When psychiatric diagnoses remain a psychiatrist's primary concern, they tend to suck all the air out of the room, reducing a patient's unique story to a lifeless coded category. When you look for the right psychiatrist, take seriously how he or she views psychiatric diagnoses. Choose a psychiatrist who understands diagnoses for what they are: rough and flawed guides, nothing more. And, most important, choose one who embraces the idea that you are more than your diagnosis.

WHY HAVE THEM?

So, if psychiatric diagnoses are so problematic, why aren't they scrapped? The short answer: money. They remain the lifeblood of mental health funding. Reimbursement depends on *DSM* codes. With all their deficiencies, psychiatric diagnoses provide a standard currency, the key to hospitals, clinics, and mental health service providers getting paid. They determine who gets treated and for how long. This is particularly true of public programs that when overloaded—as they usually are—limit services to "the most severe" diagnoses. (Ironically, such restrictions invariably exclude some of the most severely impaired patients with personality problems complicated by addiction.) One author described the *DSM* manual this way: "Though many therapists dismiss the manual as useful for only the numbered codes they scribble on reimbursement forms, it subtly permeates the consciousness of the profession. The book is required reading for almost every psychologist and psychiatrist in training. It delineates the conditions studied by researchers, and it quietly underlies our comprehension of ourselves. Its disorders define norms" (Bergner 2009).

Some will claim *DSM* diagnoses are essential to research, insisting that psychiatric studies would be impossible without reliable diagnostic criteria. But reliability, as we have seen, continues to defy *DSM* categories. And even if they were reliable, would that be enough? Criteria used by medieval witch-hunters were reliable. Very reliable. Systematically applied, they turned up numerous "witches" who met strict criteria. Reliability wasn't the problem. The problem was the faulty assumption behind the criteria. Similarly, applying *DSM* criteria to the letter—even in research settings—hardly matters if the diagnoses themselves are contrived. Psychiatric diagnoses mislead by implying "standard" problems that not all patients have while overlooking real problems that go beyond diagnoses. Like everyone else, we psychiatrists see what we look for. Once we have a category in mind, our focus narrows to observations that support it. Other aspects of the person's life fall by the wayside, until finally we arrive at the "codable" diagnosis.

The glaring flaws in *DSM* diagnoses prompted former *DSM* task force chairman Allen Frances to recommend their oversight be transferred from the American Psychiatric Association to a federal agency such as the Institute of Medicine (Frances 2012). After years of shoehorning patients into DSM categories, I now consider the exercise of questionable value, if not downright harmful. Psychiatric symptoms overlap and blend together far more than the *DSM* suggests. For the most part, I find these labels extraneous, misleading, and dehumanizing. Regardless of diagnosis, patients are individuals with their own unique combinations of symptoms, troubled stories, and life histories. Better they are understood in these terms than diagnosed.

A DIFFERENT APPROACH

Many years ago Dr. Eric Cassell wrote *The Healer's Art*, in which he distinguishes between illness and disease (Cassell 1979). A disease, he explains, is a biological breakdown; an illness, in contrast, is *how the patient experiences* his or her disease. Psychiatric diagnoses miss the boat on both counts. Failing thus far in their long-standing search to identify specific biological breakdown, too often, they also fail to take into account the patient's perception of what's happening—the sense of losing control, the struggle against hopelessness, that is, the personal meaning of the patient's situation.

Thomas Szasz once described mental illness as a myth (Szasz 1961). I disagree. If there's a myth, it's psychiatric diagnosis. Psychiatric symptoms and the problems that underlie them are *not* myths. I have seen numerous patients—out of strict adherence to "diagnosis"—inappropriately maintained on ineffective psychodrugs for years. I have watched confused patients treated for four or five different diagnoses at the same time, and I have observed diagnoses changed simply to meet "rules and regulations." What I have not seen are patients whose diagnoses were critical to their treatment. (The only exceptions being those patients with masquerading *medical conditions* whose correct medical diagnoses are essential to treatment.)

There will be those who consider my disregard for diagnosis misguided. But I ask you, what is gained by labeling a person *bipolar*? If taking lithium or some other mood stabilizer provides a patient lifesaving protection from recurrent manic episodes, by all means it should be used, regardless of whether or not the person meets criteria for bipolar disorder. Likewise, does applying the diagnosis of *schizophrenia* make a psychiatrist better able to treat recurrent "voices," delusional thoughts, and social withdrawal? I think not.

Not too long ago, the idea of *formulating* a patient's problems was common parlance. The idea was to come up with a workable explanation of a patient's symptoms and problems and a plan for productive changes. Formulation remains central to my view of clinical psychiatry. On this subject, I find the thinking of Dr. Paul McHugh, former chairman of the Johns Hopkins Department of Psychiatry, refreshing. In the book he coauthored with Phillip Slavney, *The Perspectives of Psychiatry*, he pushes for a less diagnostic, more multidimensional appraisal of psychiatric problems: "life can be altered by what a patient 'has' (disease), what a patient 'is' (dimensions), what a patient 'does' (behaviors), or what a patient 'encounters' (life stories)" (McHugh and Slavney 1998). This *perspectives framework* encourages an integrated look at various sources of personal dysfunction—biology, personality/behavior, and life story—without putting undo emphasis on any specific diagnosis. At least it's a start.

At the conclusion of his book *Before Prozac*, medical historian Edward Shorter sums up psychiatry's current plight: "Somehow, the field has lost its grip over diagnosis and therapeutics. Although other areas of medicine continue to make genuine advances in determining what is wrong with patients and treating them successfully, psychiatry is floundering in an ivory tower–spun web of diagnoses that jumble different diseases together, in a mesh of patent-protected remedies that represent, if anything, a loss of knowledge rather than a gain. This is not progress" (Shorter 2009).

With an overemphasis on diagnosis, psychiatrists risk neglecting what really matters to patients in their struggle for hope, meaning, and a sense of self-competency. Still—and I wish I could say otherwise—the chances of the *DSM* being supplanted are small to none. Given the current economics of psychiatric care, doing away with *DSM* diagnoses would prove chaotic. For the foreseeable future, psychiatrists and patients are stuck with these problematic labels. So, you want a psychiatrist who—recognizing the limitations of psychiatric diagnosis and understanding them to be more important for billing than anything else—readily finds an "approximate" *DSM* category and then puts it aside to focus on your special history, stresses, symptoms, and situation.

In the next chapter, I take a look at psychiatry's second major problem, one you should be especially aware of in your search for the right psychiatrist: the over-reliance on psychodrugs.

CHAPTER THREE

Psychiatric Medications

Their Proper Role

- Avoid the psychiatrist who views psycho-drugs as *the* treatment.

- Question the one who ignores problems for which there are no psychodrugs.

- Regardless of the psychiatrist you pick, make sure you understand the benefits and limits of psychodrugs.

- Find a psychiatrist who recognizes the risks of long-term, uninterrupted psychodrug treatment.

- If you need psychodrugs, chose a knowledge-able psychiatrist committed to the fewest number and the lowest effective dosages.

I understand the allure of psychodrugs. I have often prescribed them. For some patients they are immensely beneficial—sometimes lifesaving—but for many they have limited or no value, and they frequently cause notable side effects. Too often, they are used in place of more appropriate therapies. Even so, in certain circumstances they are essential.

My advice to you is this: whomever you choose as a psychiatrist, do not depend totally on his or her guidance regarding psychodrugs. Familiarize yourself with their legitimate uses, their potential benefits, and their adverse effects. Given the massive marketing of psychodrugs, I anticipate your surprise at what might seem overly cautious guidance. What follows likely will make you less so.

LESS THAN WHAT THEY SEEM

Modern psychodrugs first came on the scene in the early 1950s. Most of the major discoveries came by accident; and from the early 1960s onward, there would be no further advances. Two leading researchers acknowledged this puzzling lack of progress when they declared psychodrug development "at a near standstill" (Nestler and Hyman 2010). Likely, you will find this conclusion at odds with print and television ads that relentlessly portray new psychodrugs as breakthrough solutions. (I have a hard time understanding why these ads are so effective when they include, by regulation, an extensive listing of troublesome side effects that sometimes goes on as long as the promotion itself.) In truth, overall, psychodrugs are *modestly* effective; and, unlike what the ads imply, they are only *symptomatic* treatment. There are no psychodrugs for specific psychiatric disorders. There are drugs for anxiety, mania, and depression; there are no drugs for schizophrenia, autism, or bipolar disorder.

And despite the repeated promotion of new psychodrugs as "breakthrough" medications, when compared with older versions, they show no greater efficacy. The one notable exception is a drug called clozapine. Certain patients with psychosis whose symptoms do not improve on other psychodrugs respond dramatically to this medication. The reasons remain unclear. Unfortunately, the benefit is overshadowed by a cluster of *severe* side effects, including a potentially fatal condition that necessitates frequent precautionary blood checks.

Despite this lack of progress, decade after decade psychiatrists embrace glitzy announcements of "new and better" psychodrugs that are outrageously expensive. For decades bogusly heralded knockoffs have generated unseemly profits. Even more egregious, as a drug patent expiration approaches, psychodrug makers—faced with a loss of revenue—often have the gall to make minor modifications (of no clinical consequence) for the sole purpose of extending the patent with its exorbitant pricing. Protecting the franchise is everything!

I don't know which is more embarrassing: psychodrug companies marketing bogus breakthrough drugs or psychiatrists (and other physicians) blithely prescribing them as though they are valuable innovations, worth the extra cost. Throughout my career, the prescribing of psychodrugs has been a choice of *more of the same*, decade after decade. The only thing that changes are the side effects, but all psychodrugs—new or old—have them. The one clear advantage that newer antidepressants do have over the older ones relates to *lethality*. I remember well uneasy moments that arose out of prescribing the older tricyclic antidepressants for persons with severe depression, knowing full well the medication itself could be used as a suicide tool. Unfortunately, the newer antidepressants have their own set of problems.

THE SELLING OF "CHEMICAL IMBALANCE"

In the absence of any real progress, psychodrug makers have relied on marketing gimmicks (Davies 2013). By far the most successful one portrays psychodrugs as treatment for specific chemical imbalances in the brain. Since psychodrugs alter brain chemicals, so the pitch goes, the conditions they target must be caused by chemical imbalances. If a patient's depression improves after taking a serotonin-enhancing drug, the depression must be caused by low levels of brain serotonin. Similarly, if a psychosis clears after taking a dopamine-blocking drug, too much dopamine must be the culprit. A similar line of illogical reasoning would have us believe that aspirin deficiency causes headache, since when we take aspirin the headache gets better, or that pain arises from an opiate deficiency, since opiates (such as morphine) provide pain relief.

A Web advertisement for the antidepressant Paxil provides a good example of the chemical imbalance theme in action. "Just as a cake recipe requires you to use flour, sugar and baking powder in the right amounts, your brain needs a fine chemical balance in order to perform at its best" (Watters 2010). While it's true that psychodrugs cause chemical changes, likely, they do not correct chemical imbalances in the brain. This is for the simple reason that no specific chemical imbalance has been found for any psychiatric disorder (Belmaker and Agam 2008; Ongur 2009). Although psychodrugs can be quite helpful, they are purely symptomatic treatment. And it's not even clear that the symptom relief of psychodrugs stems from their reputed actions such as blocking dopamine or increasing serotonin. The brain's chemical neurotransmitters intertwine extensively. For example, a "serotonin" drug may alter dopamine levels; a norepinephrine drug may shift serotonin levels. This belies psychodrug labels like "SSRI" (selective serotonin reuptake inhibitor) or "dopamine blocker" and probably explains why improvement in psychiatric symptoms doesn't parallel changes in neurotransmitters (Khan 1999).

None of this seems to matter to psychodrug makers. They go right on promoting chemical imbalance. Clearly, it's good for business. Still, it must be a tad embarrassing when a drug such as tianeptine (sold in France and other countries) turns up. Although similar to Prozac (and other SSRI drugs alleged to *raise* serotonin levels) in efficacy, tianeptine actually *reduces* serotonin! One researcher summed it up this way: "If depression can be equally affected by drugs that increase serotonin and by drugs that decrease it, it's hard to imagine how the benefits can be due to their chemical activity" (Begley 2010). So it is not totally unexpected to find antidepressant medications that target different neurotransmitters—SSRIs, SNRIs, NaSSAs, NRIs, NDRIs—achieving the same outcomes.

In the absence of a compelling understanding of how psychodrugs work, new explanations predictably pop up. With regard to antidepressants, some researchers have suggested they exert an anti-inflammatory effect that stabilizes an overactive corticosteroid system (Barden et al. 1995). This fits with the finding that markers of an inflammatory response (cytokines) show a substantial rise in depression (Miller et al. 2009). Along the same line, a recent article—"Are Psychiatric Disorders Inflammatory-Based Conditions?"—describes how minocycline, a tetracycline antibiotic and powerful anti-inflammatory agent, improves depression (Soczynska et al. 2012). Another proposal for how antidepressants work has them promoting increased nerve cell growth, particularly in the hypothalamus (Thomas et al. 2003).

The truth is we don't know.

The same goes for other psychodrugs such as antipsychotics. For a long time psychosis (delusions and hallucinations) was considered the product of too much brain dopamine. We now know this is not the whole story. In fact there's growing suspicion that a decades-long focus on neurotransmitters and their receptors has completely missed the mark. Based on imaging studies, one researcher has posited psychosis as a breakdown in the supporting structure (white matter) of the brain (Cheung et al. 2011; Makris et al. 2010). As early as 1973, E. Fuller Torrey, with his collaborator M. Peterson, turned up evidence of a possible viral origin for schizophrenia (Torrey and Peterson 1973). Despite these intriguing speculations, the fundamental causes of psychiatric disorders remain a mystery. What we do know is this: psychodrugs do not work by correcting chemical imbalances. Even so, this powerful but misleading metaphor persists.

In your search for the right psychiatrist, look for candor. Look for someone who gives you an honest appraisal of what psychodrugs can *and* can't do instead of automatically reaching for his prescription pad.

THE GLOW IS OFF

Before I review the effectiveness of psychodrugs, we need to take a brief detour. For years psychodrugs have been touted as *significantly* better than placebo, as though this makes them particularly efficacious. Here's the problem. (Stick with me. This gets a little convoluted, but it's important.) When applied to evaluative studies, "significant" is a trick word—a statistical term masquerading as commonsense language. While implying great importance, *statistical significance* means something much less: *whatever* the outcome of a study, likely, the results—if statistically significant—did not happen by chance alone. That's it.

So, with respect to psychodrugs, being deemed *significantly* better than placebo says nothing about their overall efficacy. Tiny differences between the effects of drugs and placebo—even those of no clinical import—often qualify as *statistically significant*, the moniker of excellence required for U.S. Federal Drug Administration (FDA) approval. The FDA sets a low bar for drug approval: *two* controlled studies showing *statistical superiority* over placebo. The differences may be small, and other studies may have shown *opposite* results, but FDA approval may still be conferred! If you assume the regulation of psychodrugs (and other medications as well) is on a par with financial regulation, you will be correct. Keep this in mind and you will understand how psychodrugs continue to dominate psychiatry, despite modest results and numerous troublesome side effects.

When you look beyond the advertising at actual clinical results, psychodrugs are confusing. Your best guide is a psychiatrist who considers alternative treatments and, if you need psychodrugs, always weighs the benefits against the risks. With that said, the question remains: how effective are psychodrugs? From the outset I need to make this clear: the studies I review in trying to answer this question are based on *average* results. While providing valuable information, such results may not apply to any given individual, including you. That's why you need a psychiatrist committed to *individualized* care. I'll start with antidepressants.

Despite full-page splashy ads (and, more recently, television commercials) extolling these medications and despite their widespread use, their overall effectiveness is modest (Kirsch 2009; Davis et al. 2011). To date, the STAR* D study remains the most comprehensive appraisal of antidepressants (NIMH 2006). Over a seven-year period, approximately 2,800 patients received treatment for major depression. During the first two phases of the study, all patients took the SSRI antidepressant citalopram (Celexa) for twelve to fourteen weeks, after which those who remained depressed (or had adverse effects) were given a choice. They could switch to one of three other antidepressants— sertraline (Zoloft), bupropion-SR (Wellbutrin), or venlafaxine XR (Effexor)—or they could add to their initial medication, citalopram, one of two other drugs: the antidepressant bupropion-SR or buspirone (Buspar), an antianxiety medication thought to enhance antidepressant action. The final results were sobering.

At the study's conclusion only 56 percent of participants were free of depression, and within a year half of them had relapsed. These results are even less impressive when we assume much of the benefit represented a placebo-like response, which typically runs as high as 30–40 percent in persons with depression or anxiety. A high dropout rate was another disappointing aspect of the study: in the first phase, 21 percent; of those remaining, another 30 percent in the second phase. By the end of the study, over half the patients had dropped out. One has to assume either they did not get much relief or they could not tolerate the drug side effects. Whatever the reason, a 50 percent dropout rate raises serious questions about antidepressant medications as treatment for depression.

Keep in mind, antidepressants are the kind of medication that psychiatrist Peter Kramer, in his 1993 best-selling book *Listening to Prozac*, described as *transformative*. He insisted Prozac would usher in a new "cosmetic" psychopharmacology capable of chemically sculpting *personalities* to enhance pleasure, promote sociability, and facilitate "personal autonomy" (Kramer 1993). His was quite a vision, but the debate it sparked about the ethical implications of modifying personalities through chemistry quickly fizzled out once it became obvious that these medications barely work against depression, let alone transform personalities. In a 2002 article titled "The Emperor's New Drugs," Irving Kirsch examined the efficacy data submitted to FDA for the six most widely prescribed antidepressants approved between 1987 and 1999" (Kirsch et al. 2002). He found, based on forty-seven pharmaceutical-industry-sponsored studies of six different antidepressants—Prozac, Paxil, Zoloft, Effexor, Serzone, and Celexa—80 percent of the effectiveness was duplicated by placebo. This is a head-turning finding, particularly given that the studies were paid for by companies with a vested interest in superior outcomes. Based on Kirsch's work, *CBS 60 Minutes* recently carried a piece titled "Treating Depression: Is There a Placebo Effect?" The take-home message was simple: the average benefit of antidepressant medication is roughly equivalent to that of placebo (CBS News 2012). A similar conclusion emerged from a look at all antidepressant trials submitted to the FDA from 1987 to 2004. Half the studies showed zero benefit over placebo. Of note, this outcome was later distorted by the drug makers by the publication of cherry-picked studies giving the appearance that 94 percent of the trials were positive. In fact, only 51 percent of patients showed notable improvement (Turner et al. 2008). A more recent report documented even more unimpressive results. Antidepressants were compared with *active* placebos, which mimic drugs' side effects to make the placebos appear more credible to patients. The results suggest that antidepressant drug efficacy likely is overestimated and placebo efficacy underestimated (Moncrieff et al. 2012).

By 2010 the media had finally caught on. A *Newsweek* article— "The Depressing News About Antidepressants"—announced: "The belief that antidepressants can cure depression chemically is simply wrong" (Begley 2010). Their modest value was further documented in a subsequent *Journal of the American Medical Association* (*JAMA*) report showing these medications tend to work

only in the most severe cases. For mild to moderate depression—
the most common target of antidepressant medication—they are
no better than placebo (Fournier et al. 2010).

And even these meager results may be overstated. When
studies fail to show any advantage over placebo or when adverse
effects prove too troublesome, no problem—psychodrug makers simply throw out the results and start over. There are no
restrictions on how many studies can be done. A pharmaceutical company can keep at it until approvable results turn up.
These outcomes—no matter how difficult to come by—can
then be trumpeted as the only outcomes. (The FDA does now
require all drug studies to at least be publicly registered on a
website: www.clinicaltrials.gov.)

You might reasonably ask, Why then do antidepressants
remain so popular? One major factor relates to the tremendous influence psychodrug makers exert over psychiatric publications. In some instances these companies arrange to have
supportive articles ghostwritten! Another factor stems from
selective publication. In a review of 74 antidepressant studies,
researchers found 37 of 38 *positive* outcomes published in professional journals. In contrast, only 3 of 36 *negative* outcomes
made it into print (Turner et al. 2008). In a few instances, failed
results were buried in the report and replaced by a positive but
unrelated finding. This long-standing practice carries the nick-
name "data torturing" (Watters 2010).

Despite these unimpressive findings, I hasten to add that in
my experience sometimes these medications are extraordinarily
effective, even lifesaving. Still, as you can see, the odds are not
particularly good. You want a psychiatrist who considers antidepressant drug treatment without automatically defaulting to
its use. Not all depressed persons need an antidepressant, and
many persons who take antidepressants experience little benefit.

If your psychiatrist recommends an antidepressant and you so choose, you must be patient. Typically, it takes two to three weeks before there's improvement, and the improvement will be gradual. One unexpected benefit sometimes comes in the form of reduced anxiety. More often than not, depression and anxiety go together, and improvement in one often accompanies improvement in the other.

ANTIPSYCHOTICS: A MIXED BAG

First the good news. For the treatment of acute psychotic symptoms where a person's mind plays trick on him or her in the form of delusional thoughts or seeing/hearing/feeling things that are not present (hallucinations), antipsychotic medications can be remarkably effective (Wright et al. 2001). And, as maintenance therapy for persons recovering from acute psychosis, they also appear helpful. In the year following an acute psychotic break, persons taking these medications have less than half the risk of relapsing as those who take no medication (Leucht et al. 2012).

But there are troublesome aspects to the story as well.

The most comprehensive study of antipsychotics, CATIE (the NIMH Clinical Antipsychotic Trials of Intervention Effectiveness Study), followed 1,493 persons with schizophrenia (Lieberman et al. 2005). Each received one of five medications, four of them newer antipsychotics, one older. The most striking finding concerned dropouts. Only 24 percent finished. In other words today's standard treatment for schizophrenia— antipsychotic medication—was rejected by three out of four patients. Clearly, *sole* reliance on antipsychotic medication for persons with relapsing psychosis is unrealistic. Even so, antipsychotic medication remains the main treatment—too often, the only treatment—for these patients.

Surprisingly, the CATIE study showed the older (and much cheaper) drug to be as beneficial as the newer ones, lending support to my earlier contention that psychodrug development has not progressed in fifty years. Think of the millions of dollars spent by patients, programs, and insurance companies for newer antipsychotics based on claims that they were safer and more effective. When put to the test, neither turns out to be true. Concerning these much-ballyhooed newer antipsychotics ("atypicals" or second-generation antipsychotics—SGAs), one psychopharmacologist commented: "To put it bluntly the evidence—or rather the lack of evidence—suggests that the notion of "atypicality" has been more of a marketing concept than a pharmacological reality. . . . In brief, there is no single advantage of SGA's that has been independently replicated" (Gillman 2013).

All the drugs used in the CATIE study caused major side effects; but, contrary to expectations, the prevalence of "parkinsonian" symptoms (involuntary trembling, for example) was similar for newer and older antipsychotics. As expected, weight gain and insulin resistance were much more common among persons taking second-generation drugs (Meltzer and Bobo 2006; Swartz et al. 2008).

To be fair about it, psychodrug companies are not alone in their failure to come up with better drugs. In her hard-hitting article "The Truth About the Drug Companies," Marcia Angell, former editor of the *New England Journal of Medicine*, describes drug makers' "darkest secret": "All the public relations about innovation is meant to obscure this fact. The stream of new drugs has slowed to a trickle, and few of them are innovative in any sense of that word. Instead, the great majority are variations of oldies but goodies—'me-too' drugs" (Angell 2004). Even so, psychodrug makers are the worst offenders, having gone a half century without major breakthroughs and, even worse, acting as though they had by charging exorbitant prices.

None of this takes away from the unique benefit antipsychotic medications (old and new) provide in the treatment of acute psychotic symptoms. Their long-term use, however, is another matter, one that I consider later in this chapter (Iatrogenic Psychosis).

NEGATIVES

Many psychdrugs come to market touted as having no serious side effects, only to have this claim disproved later. All psychodrugs have adverse effects that range from bothersome to life threatening. Where previously there were dry mouth, light-headedness, shakes, and tremors, now there are major weight gain, diabetes, elevated blood lipids, and increased thoughts of suicide. Despite decades of research, psychodrug complications remain a vexing problem. The most severe complications most frequently involve antipsychotics and include neuroleptic malignant syndrome (a neurologic emergency), tardive dyskinesia (uncontrolled muscle movements that may become permanent), and disabling parkinsonian symptoms. The use of any of the antipsychotic drugs also confers higher death rates on older persons. Despite this finding, roughly one of seven nursing home patients, most of them with dementia, receive antipsychotic drugs (Harris 2011a).

There is another serious complication of antipsychotic medication that seldom receives the attention it deserves. To varying degrees all these drugs block the action of brain dopamine. Although the intricacies of how dopamine facilitates the experience of pleasure remain unknown, the central role it plays in the pleasure/reward circuitry of the brain is well established (Linden 2011). Consistent with this finding, numerous patients taking dopamine-blocking antipsychotic medications complain of feeling "empty" and exhibit a reduced capacity for pleasure. In this light, their reluctance to taking these drugs doesn't seem all that strange.

Extreme weight gain, another serious adverse effect of antipsychotics (as well as others), is so common now that mental health programs, I feel, are remiss if they don't provide fitness training as a standard service. Over an eleven-week period, 257 children and adolescents treated with second-generation antipsychotics gained, on average, 8–15 percent of their weight (Correll et al. 2009). Even more disturbing, fewer than a third of these patients had a psychotic diagnosis. This finding is consistent with what other researchers report. Stephen Crystal, a Rutgers University professor, estimates that 70 percent of atypical antipsychotic medication prescribed for children and teenagers is for nonpsychotic conditions (Wilson 2009).

Complications from psychodrugs are so common now, when one of my patients takes a turn for the worse, I immediately suspect an adverse drug effect. Newer antidepressants can cause sexual dysfunction, agitation, mania, nausea, and sleeplessness. SSRIs, specifically, appear to predispose to cataracts (Etminan et al. 2010). Mood stabilizers have been associated with pancreatitis, bleeding problems, depressed thyroid function, hepatitis, imbalance, tremors, hair loss, and various fetal abnormalities.

The weight gain associated with second-generation antipsychotics (atypicals) is often part of a larger problem known as metabolic syndrome, a condition characterized by obesity (especially in the mid and upper body), type II diabetes, high blood pressure, and increased serum triglycerides. This syndrome heightens the risk of heart disease and stroke. The four most commonly used atypicals—olanzapine (Zyprexa), aripiprazole (Abilify), quetiapine (Seroquel), and risperidone (Risperdal)—were the focus of a two-year study of 332 patients, age forty and older, with psychosis. Within one year, 36.5 percent of these patients developed metabolic syndrome. Midway through the study the exceedingly high number of serious adverse events associated with quetiapine (Seroquel) led to its discontinuation (Hua et al. 2012).

You would think psychiatrists would be keen on looking for something as serious as metabolic syndrome, but a review of forty-eight studies showed most clinicians who prescribed antipsychotics did not follow "guidelines to monitor metabolic risk" (Nasrallah 2012).

Sometimes adverse side effects to psychodrugs develop slowly. The *Huffington Post* (Internet) carried a posting by super-model, Paulina Porizkova, titled "Ending a Midlife Affair with Meds" (Porizkova 2011). She describes how after initially resisting the idea of taking a psychodrug for severe panic attacks, she eventually agreed to a prescription for Lexapro, an SSRI antidepressant/antianxiety drug. At first, she felt nothing, but with time her primary symptoms abated. "I spent two years with my lover Lexapro," she says, "the two most mellow years of my life. My immediate frustrations were comforted, my resentments muffled, my anxiety calmed; I was wrapped in a thick, warm comforter, insulated against the sharp pangs that came with living." Eventually, however, Porizkova found these comforts were coming at too great a price. "I felt emotionally Botoxed," she laments as she describes emotional distancing from her husband, children, and friends. "Life anesthetized," she calls it. So, she stopped the medication. She admits it was difficult for a while, but after ramping up her exercise routine, she returned to her normal self, happy with her decision to forgo Lexapro.

In the 1970s I was a hospital psychiatrist in Santa Clara County, California, on a unit that admitted persons with acute psychotic symptoms. Almost without exception these patients immediately were started on high doses of antipsychotic drugs, so I got a close look at various side effects. Eventually, I did something I don't recommend and probably would not do again. Convinced it would give me a better sense of what my patients were experiencing, I took a small dose of the medications I often prescribed. One morning, before rounds, I swallowed half a milligram of Haldol and one milligram of Cogentin (used with antipsychotic drugs to lessen Parkinson-like side effects). These are relatively small doses. On average, psychotic patients received ten to sixty times as much Haldol or its equivalent (sometimes more) and two to six times as much Cogentin. It took about thirty minutes for the drugs to work.

The first thing I felt was a profound sense of heaviness. Walking became labored, as though I were carrying lead in my pockets. I felt drowsy as a disquieting numbness settled over me. These uncomfortable feelings persisted for hours, but of greater concern was how the medications squashed my concentration and memory. During interviews with patients a social worker colleague, aware of what I had done, was forced to intervene. Later she told me I kept repeating myself. I do recall struggling as my attention drifted in and out. You may question my judgment in taking on this self-experiment. How much could I really learn? It's a fair criticism. Still, the experience left an indelible impression. I was never quite as cavalier about prescribing psychodrugs afterward. They truly have bothersome side effects. Too often we forget.

IATROGENIC PSYCHOSIS?

Taking psychodrugs for a limited time to control acute symptoms and prevent their immediate reoccurrence is one thing; taking them for extended periods is quite another. It's important you understand this distinction and that you find a psychiatrist who does also.

The first well-documented exposé of the detrimental effects of long-term use of antipsychotic psychodrugs was Robert Whitaker's *Mad in America* (Whitaker 2002). Whitaker is an investigative journalist by trade. He has won several national awards including the George Polk Award for medical writing and a National Association of Science Writers Award for his coverage of mental illness and the pharmaceutical industry. Originally, he set out to describe advances in psychiatric medications, but by the time he finished, he had reached a chilling conclusion: the long-term use of antipsychotic drugs appeared to leave patients more vulnerable to recurrence of psychotic symptoms than they would be otherwise.

Whitaker was not the first person to question long-term antipsychotic treatment. In the late 1970s two Canadian physicians, Guy Chouinard and Barry Jones, described tardive dyskinesia, a neurological condition characterized by involuntary jerks, twitches, and writhing movements. They concluded that most likely it was the result of extended use of antipsychotic medication that causes blocking of dopamine in brain areas (basal ganglia) essential to coordinated movement. They reasoned that the initial blockade of dopamine that characteristically caused Parkinson-like side effects led, with time, to a permanent "supersensitivity" to dopamine. The result was tardive dyskinesia, often irreversible. Today, this explanation is widely accepted.

Less well known is Chouinard and Jones's speculation that dopamine blocking might similarly cause supersensitivity in other brain areas that would make future psychotic episodes more likely (Chouinard 1980). Years later Whitaker has marshaled strong evidence for such supersensitivity psychosis. The disturbing implication is this: patients are potentially made more disabled, not less, by prolonged, uninterrupted antipsychotic treatment. Your first reaction may be disbelief. After all, we are talking about a standard psychiatric practice for chronic psychotic conditions. All I can say is this: although the incriminating clues are indirect, they are substantial and compelling. I'll summarize the findings; you decide for yourself.

One would think that psychotic persons who faithfully take antipsychotics would do better than patients who fail to take them. Certainly, this is a well-established mantra of modern psychiatry, a core assumption of mental health care. So, it's surprising to find a *1970s* report that suggests otherwise. A comparison was made of patients discharged in 1947 from the Boston Psychopathic Hospital—before psychodrugs were discovered—to those treated later with psychodrugs and discharged in 1967. Five years after leaving the hospital, 45 percent of the first group remained well as compared with only 31 percent of the psychodrug-treated group (Bockoven and Soloman 1975). An even more dramatic difference turned up in a second state hospital study. Men with schizophrenia—eighty in all— were assigned either to drug treatment or non–drug treatment and followed for three years. Of those not taking psychodrugs, 73 percent remained well. This contrasted with only 38 percent of those who took medication (Rappaport 1978).

As it turns out, these seemingly upside-down results are similar to those reported in 1964 by NIMH researchers. Initially, treatment with antipsychotics appeared quite promising. After six weeks, 75 percent of schizophrenic patients taking a psychodrug were "much or very much improved," compared with 23 percent on placebo. In fact the difference in improvement was so great, the investigators initially insisted that antipsychotic drugs be considered curative and characterized as specifically "anti-schizophrenic" in their effect. A year later, however, the initial exuberance of these same researchers disappeared after they discovered patients treated with a placebo were *less* likely to be rehospitalized (Schooler 1967). In the bloom of a new era of psychodrug treatment, these disappointing results were explained away as anomalous and quickly forgotten.

Martin Harrow, a psychologist at the University of Illinois, followed sixty-four persons with schizophrenia for fifteen years. All of them were free to take or not take antipsychotic medication. Harrow's job was simply to assess their condition periodically, noting as he went along their choice about taking medications. During a final observation, he discovered that 40 percent of persons who had refused meds had fully recovered. More than half were gainfully employed. For those who continued on medications, outcomes were not nearly as good. Only 5 percent were fully recovered; 64 percent remained actively psychotic. During this same period, Harrow also followed persons with "other psychotic disorders" including bipolar patients, severe depressives, and those with "milder psychotic conditions." They showed a similar pattern. Although, initially, bipolar persons off meds did poorly, eventually they stabilized, and at the study's conclusion they were doing better than their medicated counterparts. When Harrow ranked outcomes for all patients, the best results were achieved by manic-depressive patients *off* meds. Second best were schizophrenic patients *off* meds. Manic-depressive patients *on* meds were third, and, the least favorable outcomes occurred among schizophrenic patients *on* medications (Whitaker 2010).

More recently researchers at the University of Illinois College of Medicine published a report titled "Do All Schizophrenia Patients Need Antipsychotic Treatment Continuously throughout Their Lifetime?" Over a period of twenty years they evaluated seventy patients on six different occasions. At each of the follow-ups they found 30–40 percent no longer taking antipsychotics. These patients were less likely to be psychotic and more likely to have periods of recovery; and, despite being off antipsychotics for prolonged periods, they did not experience more frequent relapses. The researchers concluded that not all patients with schizophrenia require continuous medication throughout their lives (Harrow et al. 2012).

Admittedly, there is the possibility that these results were skewed by the fact that the most symptomatic patients were the ones who *required* medication. We can't completely rule this out. But there's an equally plausible explanation, consistent with the other studies: continuous, prolonged psychodrug treatment—currently, the gold standard for treating "chronic" psychotic conditions—is deleterious.

A second line of evidence comes from two World Health Organization (WHO) studies, the first in 1969. Outcomes for schizophrenic persons in "developed" countries were compared with those in "underdeveloped" countries. The guess was that developed countries would report superior results because of better treatment. The only real question was by how much. But the results proved otherwise. At years two and five, patients from the three poorest countries—India, Nigeria, and Colombia—fared dramatically better than patients in the United States and four other developed countries. After five years, 64 percent of patients from underdeveloped areas showed no symptoms compared with 18 percent from developed countries. These results did not play well in the United States and other richer countries. Critics questioned the study design. They criticized what they presumed was a lack of diagnostic rigor in poorer countries, suggesting that cases labeled schizophrenia most likely were milder forms of psychosis.

With this critique in mind, WHO undertook a second study in ten countries focused on patients with "first-break" schizophrenia. The results were similar. In the poorer countries 63 percent of patients had a good outcome; in the richer countries, 37 percent. No firm conclusions could be drawn as to why, but one glaring difference stood out: only 16 percent of patients in poorer countries received psychodrugs compared with 61 percent in richer countries.

A third line of evidence comes from attempts to treat acute psychosis with *minimal* psychodrugs. In the 1970s I worked in San Jose, California with the Soteria Project, a community program committed to using psychodrugs as little as possible in the treatment of early episodes of "schizophrenia spectrum psychosis." With funding from the NIMH, Soteria collaborated with the Santa Clara Valley Hospital. Psychotic patients seen at the hospital were randomly assigned either to the inpatient psychiatric unit, where I worked, or to the Soteria residential program, located in a twelve-room house in the San Jose community. While hospital treatment was primarily antipsychotic drugs, Soteria relied much more on staff-patient interaction and psychosocial therapies, using psychodrugs as little as possible. As I recall, the costs of the two approaches were about the same.

When I lost contact with the study, the results were still unknown. Several years later I was intrigued to find the two approaches had produced roughly equivalent short-term results. Longer term, however, Soteria patients fared better. They had lower relapse rates, and they showed superior results in school and work performance (Mosher 1978). Several years later, researchers conducted a similar comparison in Switzerland. The outcomes resembled those from San Jose (Ciompi et al. 1992). A 2008 review of three additional studies involving 223 participants also confirmed the original Soteria findings (Calton et al. 2008). You would think this surprising outcome likely to spur interest in minimizing the use of psychodrugs, but this has not happened. The hurdles are obvious. So ingrained is our current psychodrug-centered approach that managed care and accreditation reviewers instantly question treatment that does not emphasize medication. If the patient's condition isn't serious enough to merit medications, they reason, it is not serious enough to qualify for payment.

Although the community mental health movement of the 1970s overreached in its concern for all things social and political, it proved correct in its recognition of the essential importance of nonmedication services for persons with chronic mental problems. These patients often have life problems that extend far beyond distorted perceptions and inappropriate behavior. Today this community mental health legacy barely hangs on, overshadowed now by a preoccupation with the rebalancing of "chemical imbalance."

In most mental health programs, continuous medication is the primary—if not the only—treatment strategy for chronic mental disorder. And rarely is their any consideration of using medications intermittently. In fact, guidelines from the Schizophrenia Patient Outcomes Research Team specifically prohibit such an approach: "Strategies for targeted intermittent antipsychotic maintenance treatment should not be routinely used in place of continuous maintenance treatment due to the risk of relapse and symptom worsening" (Buchanan 2010).

As far as I know, Whitaker's basic claim remains unanswered: "there is a preponderance of evidence," he says, "showing that standard neuroleptics, over the long-term, increase the likelihood that a person will become chronically ill." I find Whitaker's contention deeply disturbing, especially in light of a similar assertion made as early as 1976 by two respected clinical psychopharmacologists. In an article titled "Maintenance Antipsychotic Therapy: Is the Cure Worse Than the Disease?" George Gardos and Jonathan Cole challenged the routine use of antipsychotic medication as maintenance treatment after they found that approximately 50 percent of patients did just as well without such treatment. "The major principle we wish to stress," they concluded, "is that every chronic schizophrenic outpatient maintained on an antipsychotic medication should have the benefit of an adequate trial without drugs" (Gardos and Cole 1976).

Recently, reduced brain volume has been associated with extended antipsychotic treatment. Researchers reported an MRI study of 211 treated patients with early-onset schizophrenia. On average, patients had three scans over the course of roughly seven years. The imaging results tied treatment with all classes of antipsychotics to decreased brain volume (Ho et al. 2011; Price 2011). While there is an ongoing debate about the significance of these brain scan results, I for one find the evidence disquieting, particularly in light of the other material I've covered here.

WEAK REBUTTAL

There are academics and researchers who think the questioning of psychodrug treatment wrongheaded, if not contemptible.

In a *New York Times* article, Dr. Jeffrey Lieberman, chairman of Psychiatry at Columbia University Medical Center and director of the New York State Psychiatric Institute, put it this way: "I am usually a pretty moderate person. But on this I am 110 percent emphatic: If the diagnosis is clear, not treating with medication is a huge mistake that risks the person's best chance at recovery. It's just flat out nuts" (Carey 2006). Others point to evidence showing that patients with chronic psychosis predictably deteriorate when they stop taking antipsychotic medication; the same for depressed patients who quit their antidepressants (Kane 2010; Kocsis 1996). Accordingly, these critics advocate continuous psychodrugs for extended periods. In many instances, for life. Some suggest that to do otherwise borders on malpractice.

What they overlook or ignore is how often patients, themselves, *abruptly* stop taking psychiatric medications. Given any degree of supersensitivity, this predictably would cause rapid relapse. In fact, a study of one thousand patients with schizophrenia showed that 50 percent of those who *suddenly* stopped their medication relapsed within thirty weeks. The rate was cut in half, however, when medication was discontinued slowly (Viguera et al. 1997). Even in instances when psychodrug dosage has been tapered, there's always the question of whether it was done slowly enough. With patients previously on high doses for long periods, extremely slow tapering may be required. Since many patients stop medications on their own, prescribing antipsychotics for chronic psychiatric conditions may well be an unwitting setup for future relapses. When seen again, such patients will likely be prescribed the same or a similar medication, and the disturbing cycle will be started again.

There is a strong belief that the longer the delay in treatment with antipsychotic medications, the poorer the outcome. But to withhold antipsychotic medication does not mean that a patient has to go without any treatment. Therapy, personal coaching, and supportive groups would be particularly appropriate for persons with no previous history of psychosis. One potential advantage of these alternatives is a lower dropout rate. In one study only 13 percent of psychotic patients stopped psychosocial treatment prematurely (Villeneuve et al. 2010). (Compare this with the massive dropout rate found in early psychodrug studies I've reviewed.) And such alternatives could always be used in conjunction with low-dose antipsychotic medication. Sadly, most treatment settings for acute psychosis provide extremely limited alternatives, if any. The substantial and disturbing case against continuous and extended use of antipsychotics has yet to influence mainstream mental health policy.

In September 2013 researchers from the Netherlands reported a seven-year follow-up of persons with first-episode psychosis. Consistent with the material I have covered, they discovered that those persons whose antipsychotic medication was minimized or discontinued relapsed at no higher rate than those maintained continuously on mediation, while achieving a level of overall functioning twice as great. In an editorial that accompanied the report of this study in *JAMA Psychiatry*, one of the researchers, Dr. Patrick McGorry, commented that the results supported the idea that "less is more" with respect to antipsychotic medication when treating these patients (Wunderink et al. 2013).

THE MYTH OF HOPELESS MADNESS

Resistance to intermittent and low-dose psychodrugs rests, in part, on the belief that any period off medication leads to inevitable deterioration. If a person suffers from an invariably catastrophic condition, why not treat him or her with continuous antipsychotics, even if they do carry risks of their own. To do otherwise is to condemn him or her to irreversible madness. This idea originated with the nineteenth-century German psychiatrist Emil Kraepelin. Without much basis, he declared schizophrenia a brain disease that invariably led to dementia. Accordingly, he came up with the first official name—*dementia praecox*. In more recent times, a similar idea was advanced by research psychiatrist and neuroscientist Dr. Richard Wyatt (now deceased). Wyatt believed that schizophrenia resulted from a neurotoxic process, which without psychodrug treatment caused progressive brain deterioration (Wyatt 1991). For years, he strongly espoused this view; but, much to his credit, when his research failed to support his belief, Wyatt issued a public retraction.

It's now clear—contrary to popular belief—that many patients diagnosed with "schizophrenia" fully recover or, at least, recover enough to live full lives—often without psychodrugs. In 1994 a psychiatric researcher reported a thirty-two-year study of schizophrenic patients discharged from the back wards of a Vermont state hospital. What she found was at great odds with today's prevailing view. Of 110 subjects, 34 percent were fully recovered and another 34 percent substantially improved (Harding 1988). Two Swiss studies turned up similar outcomes: over the long term, 50 percent of patients diagnosed with schizophrenia experienced major improvement (Ciompi 1980). The bottom line is this: too many patients labeled with "chronic mental illness" likely are being mischaracterized. The biopic movie *A Beautiful Mind* drives home the point. Following his seminal work in game theory, John Nash, while still a young

Princeton professor, fell into a severe paranoid psychosis that lasted for years. Later, however, he recovered enough to make a trip to Oslo to collect his Nobel Prize for Economics. In the 1960s Mark Vonnegut, son of the famous author, suffered several wild psychotic episodes before eventually stabilizing and going on to become a Harvard-trained primary care physician (Vonnegut 1975). Dr. Daniel Fisher had already graduated from medical school and taken up a research position at the National Institute of Mental Health when he was diagnosed with schizophrenia. Several hospitalizations later he stabilized and completed training in psychiatry. He is now codirector of the National Empowerment Center and, formerly, was a member of the president's New Freedom Commission on Mental Health.

On her way to graduating from Oxford and then Yale, Elyn Saks came down with paranoid schizophrenic and was hospitalized several times. She still hallucinates at times and on occasion finds herself delusional, particularly when she's under stress. None of this, however, has kept her from having an illustrious career. Currently, Saks is professor of law, psychology, and psychiatry at the University of Southern California and a recipient of the Catherine T. MacArthur Fellowship. In 2007 she published a *New York Times* best seller, *The Center Cannot Hold: My Journey Through Madness*, vividly describing her ongoing struggle with psychotic symptoms (Saks 2007). "High-functioning" schizophrenia is how she characterizes her problem, which she insists is not uncommon. She's married to T. R. Jones, a law professor who has been diagnosed as having bipolar disorder.

Ignore the pervasive myth that all chronic mental disorder is for always. Schizophrenia (and other "chronic" mental disorders) is not invariably for life; and, even when it persists, substantial improvement often occurs so that patients are able to lead stable, productive lives. For some, psychodrugs may never be required; for others, only intermittently; and, probably for fewer than is commonly recognized, continuously. Psychiatrists—and mental health treatment programs—often fail to make these critical distinctions. This is a serious oversight, particularly with respect to patients who might have recovered otherwise.

You want a psychiatrist who assumes all persons with mental and emotional problems are unique individuals in need of individualized treatment, regardless of diagnosis. Consider this: 5 to 7 percent of patients with schizophrenia derive no benefit whatsoever from psychodrugs. Another 10 to 25 percent relapse within six months even when taking their meds (Warner 1987). Such patients would seem ideal candidates for alternative treatments; but, more often than not, they are simply prescribed one medication after another. Presumably this is based on the firmly entrenched but misguided belief that the modern solution to all psychiatric problems is chemical. If enough psychodrugs are tried, bingo, eventually the right one will turn up. I encourage you to resist this idea. Find a psychiatrist who does the same.

KIDS ON "DRUGS"

While there are persons who greatly benefit from psychodrugs, there are others for whom psychodrugs are of questionable value and carry risks. In a recent editorial, the noted child psychiatrist Jan Fawcett described why psychiatrists are making earlier and earlier childhood psychiatric diagnoses. "We are caught in a quandary," he said, "of deciding to prescribe powerful mood stabilizers and atypical antipsychotic medications to children and adolescents with psychiatric disorders that could possibly be a detriment to their central nervous system and social development at crucial stages" (Fawcett 2010). A report by the FDA estimated that more than a half million children and adolescents take antipsychotic medication. This includes tens of thousands of preschoolers (Wilson 2010). From 2000 to 2007 there was a doubling of antipsychotic drug prescriptions for privately insured two- to five-year-olds—this despite only 40–42 percent of these preschoolers having had a mental health assessment, a single psychotherapy session, or a repeat psychiatric visit during the year they took medication (Olfson 2010a). Undoubtedly this escalation in psychodrug prescriptions will lead to more obesity and diabetes among kids.

Extended use of psychodrugs of any kind should be of concern, particularly when it involves children or adolescents. Take for example children diagnosed with ADHD. What are the risks associated with taking stimulant medications for years? Keep in mind, most of these stimulant psychodrugs have the same action as street methamphetamine. Why are psychiatrists not more concerned? Perhaps it's because of the ubiquitous chemical imbalance idea. If stimulants are simply correcting an underlying imbalance, the practice seems less draconian. Viewed from this perspective, stimulants are benign balancers, their use similar to putting oil in the car when it's low. But if we put aside the chemical imbalance myth, long-term use of stimulants appears much more ominous.

While stimulant psychodrugs often improve attention span as well as control behavior, longer-term benefits remain unproven. In truth the initial severity of ADHD symptoms and the relative social advantage of the child are far better predictors of later adjustment than is the type of treatment they receive. As for long-term complications, common sense urges caution in exposing young patients to psychoactive drugs at a time when neural pathways are rapidly developing (Poulton 2006). At a minimum, there should be demonstrated, substantial benefits in the absence of reasonable treatment alternatives.

As reported in a *New York Times* investigative article, foster children take far more than their share of psychodrugs. Often, doctors have prescribed multiple antipsychotics to control behavior in *nonpsychotic* children, resulting in frequent complications of obesity and other metabolic problems. Dr. Ramesh Raghavan, a researcher at the Washington University in St. Louis, explained this inappropriate practice: "We as a society simply haven't made the investment in psychosocial treatments, and so we are forced to rely on psychotropic drugs to carry the burden" (Carey 2011).

All in all, psychodrugs are a decidedly mixed bag. In his most recent book, *Anatomy of an Epidemic*, Whitaker summarizes his findings: "For the past twenty-five years, the psychiatric establishment has told us a false story. It told us that schizophrenia, depression, and bipolar illness are known to be brain diseases. . . . that psychiatric medications fix chemical imbalances. . . . that Prozac and the other second-generation psychotropics were much better and safer than the first-generation drugs. . . . Most important of all, the psychiatric establishment failed to tell us that the drugs worsen long-term outcomes" (Whitaker 2010).

Choose a psychiatrist who *gets* this message. It's strong stuff based on substantial evidence. Over the years, I've known numerous patients treated year after year with high doses of psychodrugs without any attempt at gradual reduction. Each time they abruptly stopped taking meds on their own, predictably, they deteriorated. Inevitably, this was taken as proof positive they needed psychodrugs forever. It's a false conclusion, especially troubling when applied to psychiatric patients for whom medications repeatedly fail to improve their overall quality of life. The medications may be what psychiatric textbooks recommend, but if they aren't doing a patient any good, they aren't worth continuing—and they may well be doing harm.

Understand, I'm not talking about patients for whom alternatives have been tried unsuccessfully and for whom psychodrugs provide unquestionable benefit. Such a patient and his or her psychiatrist are caught between the proverbial rock and hard place. But if despite treatment with several different medications, a patient fails to improve, the possibility that psychodrugs are not the answer should be considered. Regardless of diagnosis, psychodrugs don't work for many patients; and, for others, the benefit is limited compared with the risks.

PSYCHODRUGS: A PERSONAL PERSPECTIVE

Given what I've said so far, you may wonder if I see *any* value in psychodrugs. I do. In fact, some of the most valuable help I've provided patients has been the prescribing of pychodrugs for acute psychosis, panic attacks, agitation, sleeplessness, depression, obsessive thoughts, and compulsive behaviors. Used wisely, psychodrugs can provide essential temporary relief for patients in danger of being overwhelmed.

In the majority of circumstances, there are few alternatives to antipsychotic medication for the treatment of acute psychotic episodes. They are effective in chaotic situations—calming the person and lessening the disruptive quality of hallucinations and delusions—that, *sans* medication, might endanger the patient and the treatment staff. To forgo antipsychotics at such times would require much more staffing than is generally available in acute treatment settings.

Another extremely helpful class of psychodrugs are the benzodiazepines such as lorazepam and clonazepam. Despite their shady reputation for leading to addiction, these medications, appropriately prescribed, are of great value helping to control disabling anxiety. Paradoxically, they are often withheld. In some mental health clinics their use is virtually banned because of fears of addiction and medical-legal concerns. Too bad. As a short-term aid, they can be invaluable. But for sure, they need to be respected and prescribed judiciously—optimally, for persons without previous addictive problems. In a *Newsweek* article, Stevie Nicks of Fleetwood Mac fame discusses how in an effort to get her off cocaine she was started on Klonopin (clonazepam) "and the next eight years of my life were destroyed" (Nicks 2011). Benzodiazepines should be used with care, but they have a definite place in the temporary control of extreme, disabling anxiety or panic.

Based on my own clinical experience and the concerns raised by Whitaker and others, I now seriously question routine, extended use of any psychodrug, regardless of the class of medication and regardless of diagnosis *except* when experience clearly demonstrates the value of the medication and no viable alternatives. I think long-term, continuous psychodrug use appropriate only for persons who have had unsuccessful trials off medications several times following slow withdrawals. Regardless of diagnosis, psychodrugs are best used to lessen acute symptoms, and then only as long as necessary. For some, this would be a matter of hours or days; for others, weeks or months. This limited use applies even to persons with diagnoses such as schizophrenia and bipolar disorder. Recently, one of my colleagues, hearing me say this, expressed dismay. Surely I was not recommending that patients go off their medications, he questioned. He had in mind bipolar patients he had treated whose mental health he felt would have been severely jeopardized if they had stopped taking medications.

So, I want to be clear about this. I have no qualms about prescribing psychodrugs for the duration for patients who without them clearly have no chance of a reasonable quality of life or who predictably jeopardize their life, work, or family when they become psychotic. It depends on the individual, on the severity of his or her psychotic episodes, how destructive the person becomes, how well he or she tolerates medication, how significant the benefits. Psychodrugs might well turn out to be the only reasonable alternative, but not because of diagnosis alone. It's all about individualized care. But keep in mind, the majority of persons being told to stay on antipsychotics for life fail to do so. Routinely, they stop their medications in a manner that almost guarantees they will quickly relapse. In other words, the current gold standard of care is a setup. If long-term, uninterrupted treatment is what's needed, the way it's done needs to change.

Currently, uninterrupted psychodrug treatment is doled out too often simply on the basis of diagnosis. This is why no eyebrows are likely to go up if a bipolar patient stays on lithium a *dozen years* with no recurrence of symptoms. This approach fails to adequately consider risks—with respect to long-term lithium treatment, specifically, the risks of causing hypothyroidism or renal insufficiency. Surely such concerns and others I've reviewed constitute a legitimate basis for questioning *diagnostic-centered*, long-term psychodrug treatment.

Taking psychodrugs for the rest of your life is a big deal. As it is, most patients with diagnoses such as schizophrenia, bipolar, schizoaffective, and severe major depressive disorder too often are given no alternatives. You need a psychiatrist who questions established psychiatric practices driven more by diagnosis than by individual needs, a psychiatrist who will do what's necessary and best for *you*.

THE BOTTOM LINE

From long experience, I know that in certain situations psycho-drugs can be extremely effective. So, when I think they are indicated, I readily prescribe them, always being alert to side effects. My experience tells me these medications are at their best providing acute symptom relief. Higher amounts may be required initially, but I constantly try to find the lowest effective dose as a person recovers from disabling symptoms. In time I usually suggest a patient slowly taper off meds with the understanding that if symptoms return he or she can always restart them. I also emphasize the importance of being alert to signs of an impending relapse. (This is invaluable information for spouses and/or caregivers.)

Frequently, I encounter persons taking several different psychodrugs—on occasion, a half dozen or more. As a general rule, I spend time going over all of them, trying to convince both of us that there's a valid use for each one. If there's not, I explain this to the patient and with his or her permission slowly discontinue the unnecessary drugs. Sometimes this takes quite a while. Understandably, some patients feel uneasy about stopping a medication they have taken for years. In those instances

I simply keep revisiting the subject. With time, the patient usually agrees.

One of the main reasons for multiple psychiatric medications relates to their inappropriate use. It is not uncommon to see patients who have been prescribed antipsychotic medication to help them sleep! Or to keep them from feeling anxious. Question your psychiatrist about any psychodrug he prescribes so as to assure yourself that it's appropriate and essential for your problem. Take leave of the psychiatrist who won't explain the medications he or she prescribes.

Nothing I've reviewed in this chapter changes the fact that on an individual basis psychodrugs can be valuable—sometimes essential—tools. You may need them or you may not. You want a psychiatrist who will help you make that decision as opposed to concluding automatically that you have a chemical imbalance. If you have a chronic condition, you want a psychiatrist who will help you decide if extended medication is essential and, if this is the case, who recognizes the value of finding the lowest effective dose as well as exploring the possibility of closely monitored periods off medication.

Abraham Maslow, the famous humanistic psychologist, once observed: "If the only tool you have is a hammer, everything looks like a nail." If all your psychiatrist knows is chemical imbalance, prescribing psychodrugs will be what he or she does. In an article titled "The Americanization of Mental Illness," Ethan Watters laments: "The western mind, endlessly analyzed by generations of theorists and researchers, has now been reduced to a batter of chemicals we carry around in the mixing bowl of our skulls" (Watters 2010). Sadly true.

I move on to the politics of psychiatry.

CHAPTER FOUR

Psychiatrica Politicus

The Troubling Politics of Psychiatry

- Understand what you can expect from your psychiatrist under mental health law.

- Object to a psychiatrist who practices as both doctor and "jailer."

- Reject the myth that mental disability is a major cause of violence.

- Understand the insanity defense for what it is: a cynical shell game that purports to offer relief for criminal acts arising from mental disorder but gives none.

- Get angry about the relentless criminalization of the mentally disabled.

- Seek out a psychiatrist open to alternative treatments.

Of all medical specialties, psychiatry is the most politicized.

All societies try to control certain behaviors that while not illegal, cross a line: odd behaviors, bizarre, mystifying, and some- times threatening. In our particular society, since criminal law doesn't permit "preventive" detention, special mental health laws have been passed to accomplish this purpose. This is why any person assessed as mentally disordered *and* thought to be dangerous can be detained without having committed a crime.

PSYCHIATRISTS ON STAGE

"Imminent dangerousness" is the fundamental requisite for involuntary mental health treatment. Based on a cursory appraisal, a psychiatrist can order any mentally disordered per- son he or she judges to be an imminent threat to self or others detained for treatment. And, if after a short period of observa- tion, the psychiatrist continues to believe the person dangerous, he or she can petition the court to extend the incarceration. Act- ing in this role, psychiatrists—although clearly within the law— perform a task for which they have no special expertise. This fact was well established decades ago, and nothing has changed since (Cocozza and Steadman 1976).There is simply no evidence that psychiatrists (or any other mental health professionals) accurately predict imminent violence to self or others. Foren- sic psychiatric experts have compared the prediction of violence to "forcasting the weather . . . an inexact science" (Scott and Resnick 2002). What we know is this: most persons with mental problems who speak of suicide or assault do not follow through. One researcher estimates that using the best knowledge avail- able for predicting future violence, a psychiatrist will be wrong 97 times out of 100 (Szmukler 2001). Another commentator has

estimated that roughly five thousand noncriminal mentally disordered persons deemed potentially dangerous would have to
be detained to prevent one homicide (Crawford 2000).

In short, we psychiatrists play a *fictional* role in mental health
law. Without demonstrated violence-predicting expertise, we
declare patients dangerous to themselves or others. Courts routinely accept this "expert" declaration as grounds for involuntary confinement. In addition, as a result of this questionable
arrangement, what should be a straightforward doctor/patient
relationship becomes adversarial: the psychiatrist's quasi-legal
role compromises his or her legitimacy as healer. I admit to having signed numerous petitions for involuntary confinement and
having appeared in court in support of forced hospitalization
and treatment. But this dual assignment has always bothered
me. Over time, I've come to view it as inappropriate and completely unnecessary.

Other aspects of the mental health law—its procedures and
hearings—are often more pretense than real. Patients detained
as "dangerous" typically spend little time with their lawyers
(most of whom are court appointed). I've actually been asked
by patients' defense counsel to fill them in on the story even
though I was the psychiatrist advocating involuntary detention.
Seldom have I run into sharp legal advocacy for mental health
patients. There is much "winking" and "nodding" in these procedures. I have practiced in settings where, even if a patient
agrees to remain hospitalized, the official status remains "involuntary" just in case the patient changes his or her mind.

If you find yourself in a situation where your psychiatrist
is doing double duty, holding you against your will and trying
to treat you at the same time, you have the right to expect your
release as soon as you have established that you are in control

and do not represent a danger to yourself or others. Mental health laws allow your involuntary detention only as long as you remain an imminent danger as reflected in the ways you speak and behave. During the time you are held, you have the right to be actively treated for your alleged mental problem. In addition I would encourage you to ask for a different psychiatrist, one who is not both your "jailer" and your treating physician.

For what it's worth, this is my take on involuntary mental health treatment. If decisions can't be made without the pretense of psychiatric crystal-ball gazing, mental health laws should be rewritten. Given that mental health professionals cannot accurately predict violence stemming from mental disturbances, such speculation should be eliminated as a deciding factor. Instead, the laws should insist that such decisions be rendered on a *commonsense basis* by agents of the court whose responsibility it is to decide if a patient meets the *legal* requirements for involuntary detention. Police routinely do this when they bring mental patients to emergency rooms or to psychiatric facilities. Other court representatives can do the same.

Undoubtedly, there will be those who question this approach. What about psychiatric assessment? Surely a specific diagnosis must be rendered. To the contrary, mental health laws typically require only the generic assertion that a person suffers from a mental/emotional problem. Commonsense decisions about forced temporary treatment under the law will be no more difficult than decisions made every day by judges and juries. These determinations should be handled expeditiously twenty-four hours a day by duly appointed and trained agents of the court—not by psychiatrists or other mental health professionals.

At the present time, absent such agents of the court, psychiatrists should avoid, as much as possible, the mixed role of healer and jailer. The only special expertise we bring to decisions about involuntary treatment resides in our signatures. Nothing I've said, however, implies that a psychiatrist should not voice an opinion when he or she strongly feels someone is dangerous to himself or others. Such *opinion* would become part of a larger body of evidence gathered by persons responsible for seeing that a decision regarding involuntary treatment is rendered justly.

As someone trying to find the right psychiatrist, you should be aware of how the current arrangement complicates the psychiatrist's therapeutic role. No matter how competent and well meaning your psychiatrist, your interest and society's interest may conflict. At a minimum, you need to recognize the split allegiance psychiatrists are forced to assume (Greenberg and Shuman 1997). Every day thousands of patients in this country fall under the care of psychiatrists who awkwardly serve as both jailer and healer.

FACTS ABOUT MENTAL DISABILITY AND VIOLENCE

Reading between the lines, the existence of mental health laws implies that mentally disabled persons are more likely to become violent than the rest of us. This reflects a strongly held public misconception. Despite frequent public pronouncements to the contrary, persons most prone to violence are not the mentally disabled. This dubious distinction goes to young males of lower intelligence and socioeconomic status with histories of violence, physical abuse, and addiction (Scott 2005). On average psychiatric patients are no more violent than the general population. Of all persons with mental problems, the National Institute of Mental Health estimates 7.7 million suffer severe illnesses in the form of schizophrenia, schizoaffective disorder, and bipolar disorder. Of these persons, only about 1 percent (77,000) commit violent and other lawbreaking actions (Torrey 2013). Although these cases cannot be ignored, the figures illustrate the relative *infrequency* of violence among mentally disabled persons.

Sensational media coverage of crimes that psychologically disturbed persons sometimes enact obscures the relative rarity of such acts. When such persons (particularly those who are psychotically paranoid) commit violent crimes, it is not unexpected to find them "irrational," "bizarre," "crazed," or "grotesque," reflecting the deeply disturbed thought of such individuals. Evidence does suggest that a notable fraction of mass murders are committed by severely mentally disturbed persons (Torrey 2014). When these events happen, bold, oversize headlines and twenty-four-hour media coverage unwittingly promote the idea that everyone with mental disability is potentially violent and to be feared (Monahan 1997). The truth is only 3–5 percent of all violent crime is committed by persons with mental disabilities (Friedman 2006).

The authors of the 1992–1995 MacArthur Foundation study of violence committed by persons discharged from psychiatric facilities summarized their findings this way: "violence risk attributed to people with mental disorders vastly exceeds the actual risk presented. Indeed, for people who don't abuse alcohol and drugs, there is no reason to anticipate that they present greater risk than their neighbors. . . . Violence in this population only rarely results in serious injury or death and generally does not involve the use of weapons. People with mental disorders are less likely [than the general population] . . . to assault strangers and to commit assaults in public places" (Torrey et al. 2008).

Much of my clinical work has been done on acute psychiatric units. Over a period of several decades, only one patient has ever struck me. A muscular, angry man, intensely paranoid, gave me a slap on the back of the head, delivered after he had endured a series of forced medication injections. I don't mean to imply that psychiatrists or others should not be alert to the possibility of violence, particularly when caring for someone who is severely paranoid and has been psychotically violent in the past. Even so, the blanket assertion that mentally disabled persons are high risk for violence is more prejudicial than factual. Compare the way our society deals with mentally disabled persons and those persons who abuse substances. Short of flagrant intoxications, seldom are persons who drink or drug excessively detained—this despite their statistically much greater likelihood of becoming violent. Any attempt to do otherwise would meet with strong protests, and understandably so: after all, how many drinks or drug hits a day would it take to merit preventive detention? And where would it stop; what other potentially violent or self-injurious behaviors should be considered? How about riding motorcycles? NASCAR racing? Skydiving? Speeding? Several rounds of drinks?

To be sure, there are those who insist preventive detention for mentally disabled persons is different. They claim that because these persons suffer from a special kind of impaired judgment (lack of insight), they are unable to recognize their need for treatment. Accordingly, forced intervention becomes necessary *and* justified. What appears to be a compelling argument, upon closer scrutiny, however, seems less so when you realize how selectively it's being applied. Certainly mentally disabled persons have no corner on denial or impaired judgment. Persons engaged in excessively risky or criminal behavior characteristically deny the problematic nature of what they do. But of the rather large population of persons who break societal rules, it's only the mentally disabled who are targeted for preventive detention and saddled with the stereotype of forever being on the verge of attacking anyone around them. If you suffer from a mental disorder, you should be aware of the considerable exaggerations in the media and inconsistencies in the law regarding your potential for violence.

INSANITY DEFENSE AS SHELL GAME

Like predictions of dangerousness, much psychiatric court testimony is unsupported by special expertise. In matters pertaining to a person's mind at the time of an alleged crime, the only thing psychiatrists (or psychologists) have to offer is speculation. We have no legitimate expertise that enables us to reconstruct mental states from the past (Winslade and Ross 1983). With respect to the insanity defense, the psychiatrist's role becomes even more problematic because of the duplicity of the law itself. Theoretically, this legal defense provides protection against a person's being punished for criminal acts arising from mental illness; in reality, it does nothing of the sort. This is because "insanity," contrary to what you might think, is a legal—not psychiatric or medical—term. Completely divorced from the major psychotic thought distortions of severe mental disability, the legal definition of insanity reduces the insanity defense to ashes.

In practice, the defense operates like the old bait-and-switch con. Established presumably as a legal safeguard, it is then so narrowly defined as to hardly ever apply. This jaded legal maneuver creates the likelihood that persons who commit crimes in response to psychotic delusional beliefs will *not* be found insane. For this reason many mentally disabled persons accused of crime are advised by their lawyers not to use the defense. Even when a person wracked by psychotic delusions becomes fully convinced that criminal behavior is necessary and justified to protect his or her life or the lives of loved ones, more likely than not, if he or she acts on this belief, the insanity defense will provide no relief. In the eyes of the law, only one thing matters: did the person, at the time of the alleged crime, understand that what he or she was doing was wrong or, at least, that it would be considered wrong by society. If the answer is yes, an insanity defense will prove to be worthless. The severity of the person's mental derangement and its role in the crime will be deemed of no legal consequence.

In times past the insanity defense was more broadly defined, taking into account the powerfully distorting effect of psychosis on human perception and behavior. But this is no longer true (Bonnie et al. 2000). Let me illustrate this with a hypothetical case. A man with severe paranoid delusions becomes convinced that alien creatures threaten not only his own life but the lives of his daughter and granddaughters. There is no question in his mind that this is true. A compelling, godlike "voice" has told him so. In time the voice convinces the man he must act if he and his family are to avoid unspeakable torture and death. The voice directs him to destroy the aliens' secret energy supply hidden under the local twenty-four-hour convenience store. So, to save himself and his family, in the early hours one morning this terrified, deluded man sets fire to the store, knowing full well that arson is wrong and not the way he has been taught, but feeling it is his only way out. Tragically, an unsuspecting employee, trapped inside, dies. A few days later, the psychotic arsonist turns himself in to the police.

Under prevailing insanity laws, this man would be judged crazed but *not* insane. His belief that his act of arson was a matter of life or death would prove to be of little consequence given the law's narrow definition of insanity: failing to know the difference between right and wrong. In the eyes of the law, the man's awareness that it's "wrong" to burn down buildings proves his sanity.

Much of the public believes the insanity defense a giant loophole, abused mainly by hardened criminals to escape punishment they deserve. Convinced of this, the Nixon administration, in it its war on crime, considered having the law repealed as a way of keeping criminals from gaming the system and avoiding responsibility. One study found that, on average, persons queried about the insanity defense guessed it was used in more than a third of felony cases and was successful half the time. In Wyoming, from 1970 to 1972 (a time during which only one accused felon successfully pled insanity), state politicians were asked to estimate the success of the defense. They guessed 40 percent (Lilienfeld et al. 2010). Way off. The insanity defense is used in fewer than 1 percent of applicable cases; and, even then, usually, it's unsuccessful. And of the tiny percentage of defendants who are declared legally insane, only 15 percent ever go free. On average they spend thirty-three months in a locked psychiatric hospital. Typically, although found not guilty (by reason of insanity), these persons remain in institutions as long as criminals convicted of the same crimes stay in prison (Lilienfeld et al. 2010).

I choose my words carefully here: the insanity defense is a *sham*. Posing as relief for those who commit crimes because of mental derangement, this defense accomplishes the opposite by excluding any realistic consideration of the devastating impact of acute psychosis on normal behavior. The insanity defense is a legal pretense, designed mainly to ensure that mental derangement will have its day in court but rarely be accepted as a complete defense. Those few instances where it does "succeed" are almost always plea agreements. The prosecutor agrees to a finding of insanity with the proviso that the person stays in a mental hospital for years if not for the rest of his or her life. If you suffer from a mental disorder, you should be aware of the hollowness of the insanity defense. It ensures that the law, even though it says otherwise, will seldom find mental disorder an acceptable defense against criminal behavior.

JAILS FOR HOSPITALS

No doubt the absence of a realistic insanity defense contributes to the relentless incarceration of mentally disabled persons. In May of 2010 the Treatment Advocacy Center detailed where it is that mentally disabled persons actually receive their treatment. A team of law enforcement and mental health professionals found three times as many seriously mentally disabled persons treated in jails and prisons than in hospitals. Three of our country's largest providers of public mental health "care" are not hospitals; they are jails (Cook County, Los Angeles County, and Riker Island). Given the dramatic drop in psychiatric beds at hospitals—tenfold between 1955 and 2005—this development is not all that surprising. In 1955 there was one psychiatric bed for every three hundred Americans; by 2005, one for every three thousand (Torrey et al. 2010). With the closure of state mental care hospitals in the 1960s and 1970s under the banner of "least restrictive treatment," federal funds for community mental health dried up. Local resources proved grossly inadequate. Thousands of patients became homeless and ended up on the streets. It was only a matter of time before jails and prisons became the solution. Today, this jaded transfer of psychiatric care to jails and prisons continues unabated. But it's such a blatantly inappropriate response even law enforcement is speaking out. On February 13, 2012, a local television broadcast out of Akron, Ohio, announced the local sheriff's decision to stop accepting prisoners with mental illness into the jail. The decision was made after an inmate with bipolar disorder died in a confrontation with deputies. The sheriff was quoted as saying: "The indigently mentally ill in Summit County—their treatment is barbaric. We are putting them in cells. If they get out of line, we strap them in four point restraints and we leave them in there. . . . that's the way they treated them 400 years ago, and yet we're still treating them that way" (Shea 2012).

The criminalization of mentally ill persons continues despite evidence that alternative interventions produce far better outcomes. Parents across the country struggle at home with out-of-control children who need mental health care but cannot get it until eventually the children cross the line, become violent, and enter the criminal justice system. In those rare instances where they get a second chance at mental health care through mental health courts (dedicated to problem solving as opposed to punishment), they often do remarkably well. In a 2010 article titled "Effect of Mental Health Courts on Arrests and Jail Days," researchers described one thousand patients seen in mental health courts for various criminal activities. Over eighteen months those treated in lieu of being locked up recorded far fewer arrests and fewer days in jail (Steadman et al. 2010).

If you suffer from chronic mental illness, likely, you are already familiar with what I've been saying. And, you probably understand that the belief that mental disability equates with violence is only one aspect of a larger, stigmatizing myth that goes something like this: mentally ill persons, weak of character and lazy, do not deserve special help. A stronger version portrays them as straight-out deadbeats, potentially violent, who feign mental problems in order to duck responsibility, elicit sympathy, or obtain financial help. The implications are clear: beyond the demands of political correctness, mentally disabled persons deserve no special favors.

PUSHING PSYCHODRUGS

When it comes to the domination of psychodrugs in psychiatry, we are talking about a different kind of politics. Financial politics. Of the various therapies available to psychiatrists, psychodrugs overwhelmingly dominate, not (as we have seen) because of their outstanding results, but because of the influence psychodrug companies exert—financial clout that is the lifeblood of psychiatric research, publications, and education. The influence of psychodrug companies extends even into consumer groups. A *New York Times* obituary for Harriet Shetler, a founder of the National Alliance for the Mentally Ill (NAMI)—an organization one former NIMH official described as "the greatest single advocacy force in mental health"—reported that psychodrug makers contributed almost $23 million to the Alliance, representing 75 percent of all its donations (Martin 2010).

As part of their marketing strategies, psychodrug makers push certain psychiatric diagnoses. If you doubt this, read Shannon Brownlee's account of SmithKline's masterful 1990s selling of "social anxiety disorder" as a way of marketing Paxil (Brownlee 2007). Or catch another version of the same story in Ethan Watters's intriguing book *Crazy Like Us: The Globalization of the American Psyche* (Watters 2010). None of this is too surprising. These companies have one main obligation—making money for their shareholders. Marketing and research targets this goal much more than it does turning out superior psychodrugs. In some parts of our economy, markets are competitive enough so that best values for consumers emerge along with good profits. Not so when it comes to psychodrugs. For decades, drugmakers have generated phenomenal profits by producing "me-too" drugs that provide no additional benefit.

When you look for a psychiatrist, keep this background information in mind. The core training of most practicing psychiatrists has emphasized psychodrugs. You want to assure yourself that your psychiatrist has accumulated more tools in his tool kit than just psychodrugs. If so, he or she has managed to escape considerable pressure to do otherwise.

NUTRITION SUPPLEMENTS AND EXERCISE AS ALTERNATIVES

Because they are not patentable, alternatives to psychodrugs are of little interest to psychodrug makers. Accordingly, they make few if any funds available to researchers to explore this subject. This is why there are relatively few published studies on the efficacy of alternative psychiatric treatments. Even so, if a psychiatrist is willing to search for it, he or she will find evidence that alternative treatments are sometimes as effective, if not more so, than prescription psychodrugs. I offer the following as a mere sampling of findings regarding two alternative treatments: nutritional supplements and exercise. (If you are interested in more on this topic, check out the alternative medicine NIH website, www.NIH.NCCAM.gov, and the Stanley Medical Research Institute website, www.stanleyresearch.org.)

I'll start with nutritional supplements.

Abundant in fish oil, the health food supplement, omega-3 fatty acid has long been recommended as a treatment for elevated triglyceride levels. Less well known is its value in treating depression (Wolkowitz et al. 1999; Su et al. 2003; Mischoulon et al. 2009). Head-to-head comparisons show omega-3 fatty acid equal in efficacy to antidepressants such as Prozac (Jazayeri et al. 2008). This benefit extends to depressed children (Nemets et al. 2006). A plausible case can be made for using this supplement to treat mild-to-moderate depression (keep in mind, this is the form of depression for which antidepressants provide no benefit over placebo). And, given its superior side-effect profile, omega-3 fatty acid might well play a valuable role in the treatment of depressed pregnant women.

But there's more to the story. This same supplement has also proven helpful in psychotic conditions. In a twelve-week trial, patients taking supplemental omega-3 fatty acid showed improvement across the board, for both positive and negative symptoms (Peet 2001). More recently, Austrian researchers identified what they considered a *protective* effect. In a study of eighty-one patients at risk for schizophrenia (ages thirteen to twenty-five), treatment with 1,200 milligrams daily of omega-3 fatty acid was compared with a placebo (coconut oil). One year later, only 5 percent of those persons taking omega-3 fatty acid were psychotic as compared with 28 percent on placebo. Moreover, none of the persons on omega-3 supplements experienced sexual dysfunction, weight gain, or metabolic change.

The only adverse finding was mild gastrointestinal complaints (Amminger et al. 2010). Compared with psychodrugs (especially those still under patent protection), omega-3 fatty acid is inexpensive, which, ironically, means less incentive for profit-seeking drug developers to research and better establish its therapeutic benefits. As a consequence, omega-3 fatty acid likely will remain a fringe alternative, outside mainstream psychiatric treatment.

Other supplements also show promise. For example, magnesium, commonly deficient in the American diet and susceptible to depletion by stress, seems to counteract depression. One report documented depressed persons recovering after taking extra magnesium (125–300 mg) with each meal and at bedtime. When put to the test, magnesium also exerts a mood-stabilizing effect, which may be related to chemical characteristics shared with lithium (Eby 2006).

For years alternative medicine practitioners touted the amino acid tryptophan (a precursor of serotonin) for depression. But in 1989, following a mysterious outbreak of eosinophilia myalgia, the FDA removed it from the market. (Later, this problem was traced to a single batch of contaminated tryptophan shipped from Japan.) Despite its proven safety in baby food formulas, intravenous feeding solutions, and veterinary products, the FDA has yet to reapprove tryptophan. Luckily, there is a readily available substitute: 5-hydroxytyptophan (5-HTP), a chemical precursor of serotonin. In a comparison with the SSRI fluvoxamine, 5-HTP-treated patients had better outcomes and fewer adverse effects (Poeldinger 1991). In another study a group of patients *successfully* treated with an SSRI antidepressant were switched to a low-tryptophan diet. Within a short time they became depressed again. When tryptophan was reintroduced, the patients quickly recovered (Risch and Nemeroff 1992).

Both inositol and folic acid also appear to have antidepressant action. As a naturally occurring variant of glucose, inositol plays an essential role in the action of various neurotransmitters and hormones. As an alternative to standard psychodrugs inositol has shown promise in depression, panic attacks, and obsessive-compulsive behavior (Levine 1997). Compared with most psychodrugs, this supplement is extremely well tolerated and very cheap.

Augmentation is a common psychodrug strategy. When an initial psychodrug fails to work (or proves to be only partly effective), another drug is added in an attempt to improve the outcome. Folic acid improves the effectiveness of prescription antidepressants and the mood stabilizer valproate (Coppen and Bailey 2000; Behzadi et al. 2009). Several anecdotal reports suggest the efficacy of folic acid as sole treatment for depression (Stahl 2010).

Found throughout the body, the methyl donor SAMe (S-adenosyl methionine) plays a key role regulating various hormones and neurotransmitters. A Harvard Medical School/ Massachusetts General Hospital study focused on patients who despite taking antidepressant medication for some time remained depressed. During a subsequent six-week period, each patient received additional SAMe (800 mg) or a placebo. Patients on SAMe benefited twice as much and exhibited a much higher rate of complete remission: 25.8 percent versus 11.7 percent. A more recent review found SAMe, as with folate, an effective and well-tolerated *single* therapy for depression (Papakostas et al. 2012).

Gamma-amino-butyric acid (GABA) serves as a neurotransmitter essential to (among other actions) muscle relaxation. Brain concentrations increase after a person consumes the amino acid N-acetylcysteine (NAC), commonly found in nuts and seeds. In 2007, the *American Journal of Psychiatry* carried an article documenting reduced cocaine craving in addicts treated with NAC (LaRowe et al. 2007). A second study showed NAC supplementation reduced the urge to gamble three times as much as placebo (Grant et al. 2007). Notoriously difficult to treat, another form of compulsive behavior, trichotillomania (the irrational desire to pull out one's hair), also responds to NAC. In one study, half of patients given NAC experienced 50 percent or greater reduction in hair loss compared with no improvement in the control group. Remarkably, none of the patients taking NAC reported adverse effects (Grant et al. 2009). NAC also appears to improve obsessive nail biting, negative symptoms of schizophrenia, and depression in bipolar persons (Berk et al. 2009). The supplement is widely available in health food stores.

And then there's caffeine.

Stanford psychiatry professor Lorrin Koran and his research team studied the addition of a stimulant drug to the treatment regimen of persons with severe obsessive-compulsive symptoms. While continuing their previously prescribed SSRI, patients took, in addition, one of two stimulants: dextroamphetamine or caffeine. The researchers were surprised when caffeine (used as the control) produced improvement equal to that achieved with dextroamphetamine. In addition, caffeine was associated with an unexpected *reduction* in anxiety (Koran et al. 2009).

Further evidence of caffeine's therapeutic value comes from a study of fifty thousand women. Those who drank two to three cups of coffee a day were 15 percent less likely to require treatment for depression over a ten-year follow-up period (Lucas et al. 2011). The results suggest that increasing one's consumption of caffeine might help stave off depression in persons so predisposed.

Even aspirin has shown promise for certain psychiatric symptoms.

In a study funded by the Stanley Medical Research Institute, persons with schizophrenia spectrum diagnoses who were taking antipsychotic medication added either a placebo or 1,000 mg per day aspirin. After three months, those on daily aspirin had fewer symptoms. Interestingly, improvement was most pronounced in patients with the highest levels of inflammatory biomarkers (Laan et al. 2010). Aspirin, as is well known, induces a powerful anti-inflammatory response.

And how about red clover? Definitely something your psychiatrist likely will not read about in standard psychiatric journals. With a goal of testing red clover extract on depression and anxiety, Austrian researchers followed a group of postmenopausal women. After ninety days, those taking red clover reported a notable lessening of both symptoms—roughly 75 percent improvement compared with 21 percent in the placebo group (Lipovac 2010.)

But don't misunderstand me. I don't mean to portray alternative supplement treatments as a panacea. As with psychodrugs, the alternative medicine field is replete with over-the-top, bogus claims, most of them based purely on anecdotal evidence, and some nutritional supplements have serious side effects. Several years ago I authored a book titled *Health Fact, Health Fiction* that explored the subject of inflated treatment claims, which I termed "health hype" (Taylor 1990). Many alternative medicine remedies turn out to be prime examples. So, let me make it clear: I am not suggesting you seek out a psychiatrist who adopts alternative treatments carte blanche; rather, given the meager, across-the-board results of psychodrugs and their growing list of adverse effects, I recommend you find a psychiatrist *open* to trying cheaper and safer treatment alternatives. For certain, your psychiatrist will have to search beyond traditional psychiatric journals and pharmaceutical-sponsored symposia. Eventually, any decisions about alternative treatments should be based on the best information available along with his or her own clinical experience (Lake and Spiegel 2007). Above all your psychiatrist should be convinced that any prescribed alternative treatment has a good possibility of working and has tolerable risks for you.

MOVING MUSCLES VERSUS TAKING PILLS

The suppressive influence of psychodrug makers extends beyond nutritional supplements. Despite numerous studies documenting the mental benefits of exercise, they are reported infrequently in psychiatric journals. Exercise appears to improve chronic fatigue, depression, panic disorder, premenstrual dysphoria, psychotic symptoms, and substance abuse (Konstantinidou and Dratcu 2006). In his book *Spark: The Revolutionary New Science of Exercise and the Brain*, Harvard clinical associate psychiatrist John Ratey provides an overview that includes more than seventy reports detailing how psychiatric symptoms improved with exercise. In one study patients engaging in weekly, high-intensity exercise (burning 1,400 calories— 8 calories per pound), experienced, on average, a 50 percent decrease in depression. The intensity of exercise was critical. A low-intensity group (burning 560 calories—3 calories per pound) showed less improvement (33 percent), similar to that experienced by persons participating in a stretching group (Ratey 2008).

So how does exercise stack up against antidepressant medication? One four-month trial made a direct comparison. Led by Dr. James Blumenthal, Duke researchers divided 156 older patients into three treatment groups: sertraline (SSRI), exercise, and a combination of the two (Blumenthal et al. 1999). The exercise component consisted of supervised walking or jogging at 70–85 percent of aerobic capacity for thirty minutes three times a week. All three groups showed major reductions in depressive symptoms, and half went into complete remission. Over the long run, however, exercise proved superior. After six months, only 8 percent of exercisers had relapsed, compared with 38 percent of the sertraline group and 31 percent of the combined treatment group (Babyak et al. 2000). Commenting on this outcome, Ratey said: "The results should be taught in medical school and driven home with health insurance companies and posted on the bulletin boards of every nursing home in the country, where nearly a fifth of the residents have depression" (Ratey 2008).

Exercise also benefits persons with panic attacks. German researchers compared the antidepressant clomipramine to exercise. After ten weeks, both treatments were associated with fewer panic episodes. Surprisingly, the exercise group had the greatest number of dropouts: 31 percent, compared with placebo, 27 percent, and clomipramine, 0 percent (Broocks et al. 1998).

Under the direction of Harvard psychiatrist George Valliant, researchers have worked for decades to identify human experiences associated with "the good life." As it turns out, regular exercise strongly correlates with late-life mental health. In fact, it is a better predictor of future mental health than it is of future physical health (Shenk 2009). These researchers have also found that six months of moderate aerobic activity improves cognitive function in older persons (Erickson and Dramer 2009).

Ratey relates how when he approached the American Psychiatric Association about adding exercise to its official list of treatment options for depression, he was told: No deal. Not enough "scientific evidence." In the shadow of "chemical imbalance," exercise remains a difficult sale. From personal experience, I can assure you, it's much easier to get consumers to take psychodrugs than it is to get them to exercise regularly!

The politics of mental health and psychiatry run deep. As a patient trying to find the right psychiatrist, take this to heart: don't settle for less than someone who will rise above the politics as your interests demand. Also keep in mind the very real, persisting stigma attached to mental disorder and those who suffer with it. This is a deep-seated social bias. Although there are laws designed to prevent discrimination against mentally ill persons, they are not foolproof. Too often, psychiatric diagnoses become undeserved barriers to employment and other pursuits. Unfortunately, full disclosure about your psychiatric problems and psychiatric treatment—despite what you may be told—is not always in your best interest.

In the next chapter, I take up the interplay of mind, brain, and body. Given psychiatrists' combined medical and psychological training, this is an area where they should shine. Sadly, more often than not, such is not the case.

CHAPTER FIVE

Mind and Body

Psychiatrists' Rightful Place

- Don't trust a psychiatrist who insists psychiatry is a brain science.

- Make certain your psychiatrist understands both mindful and biological explanations.

- Choose one who is alert to possible medical causes of your "psychiatric symptoms."

- Find a psychiatrist who embraces the interplay between mind and brain/body.

Despite great advances in our understanding of the brain and how it works, the mind remains the life we know but don't understand scientifically. It's where we live, the setting for our life stories, the place where we experience joys, challenges, and defeats. There is no question that mind, brain, and body influence one another in powerful ways. Choose a psychiatrist who remains a competent physician comfortable working holistically.

NEUROSCIENCE HYPE

As we learn more about how the brain, genome, and experience interact, likely there will be definite neuroscience payoffs for psychiatry. Some psychiatrists are convinced this is just around the corner. Take for example UCLA psychiatrist Dr. David Fogelson: "We are poised to make dramatic breakthroughs . . . using techniques that are borrowed from molecular biology, genomic research, neuroanatomy, basic cognitive neuroscience, brain imaging, and psychopharmacology research . . . integrated with clinical data as codified in DSM-IV" (Fogelson 2010). Dr. Henry Nasrallah, editor in chief of *Current Psychiatry*, voices a similar opinion when he insists psychiatry's future "is bright because it is intimately linked to neuroscience discoveries, which ultimately will delineate specific brain path ways underlying psychiatric nosology and treatment" (Nasrallah 2010). As you read further, however, Dr. Nasrallah acknowledges that psychiatric diagnoses exhibit "far more reliability than validity" and that our understanding of how psychodrugs work is based more on "serendipity" than "evidence-based neurobiologic mechanisms." Eventually, it becomes obvious that Nasrallah is only *hoping* that brain science breakthroughs will rescue psychiatry.

Keep this in mind: over and over again, predictions of psychiatry becoming a brain science have failed to materialize. We weren't far into the age of the genome before behavioral genetics was declared psychiatry's next frontier. But after numerous studies and millions of research funds, no one has linked specific genes to psychiatric conditions. The search for the genetic origins of psychiatric disorders has been a bust (Verweij et al. 2010). The truth is, remarkably little science backs current clinical psychiatry. Neuroscience discoveries break out all around us but fail to translate into useful clinical psychiatric tools. This has been true for decades, and there is no reason to think it's about to change anytime soon. Clinical psychiatrists are not brain scientists.

One serious unintended consequence of this perennial false faith in a psychiatric neuroscience is neglect of the world of mind. Many brain scientists consider mind a quaint if not silly concept. Ultimately, it's all brain, they contend; the mind is *imaginary*. Francis Crick, the codiscoverer of the structure of DNA and later cognitive science researcher, says it this way: "You, your joys and your sorrows, your sense of personal identity and free will, are in fact no more than the behavior of a vast assembly of nerve cells. . . . You're nothing but a pack of neurons" (Horgan 1999). In their infatuation with chemical imbalance, many psychiatrists fall into this camp, believing that human passions, derangements, and satisfactions are best understood biochemically. No need for references to mind, which after all is only a shadowy illusion. No need to try and make narrative sense of personal problems. Only the biology matters.

Eric Kandel, psychiatrist, neuroscientist, and Nobel Prize winner, advocates "a new intellectual framework for psychiatry" (Kandel 1998). "All functions of mind reflect functions of the brain," he insists, so "behavioral disorders that characterize psychiatric illnesses are disturbances of brain function." In other words, mind problems are nothing more than a mirage. This worldview may be fine for neuroscientists, but it's paralyzing for clinical psychiatrists.

The cover of a recent issue of *Science Illustrated* carried the image of a surreal-looking, blue-tinted brain overlaid with the words "The Brain Explorers" (*Science Illustrated* 2010). The subtitle read, "Inside the Cutting-Edge Quest to Map the Human

Mind." Too often brain scientists equate mind with neurons, neurotransmitters, and neuroreceptors. They are way ahead of themselves. Nobel physicist Eugene Wigner got it right four decades ago when he noted: "We have at present not even the vaguest idea how to connect the physio-chemical processes with the state of mind" (Wigner 1969). Little has changed.

There is simply no compelling biological explanation for the workings of the mind. What we do know from daily experience is this: mind and brain are categorically different, so different we are forced to use separate languages to describe them. We can't reasonably explain the mind in the same words we use to describe brain/body. Note, I'm not talking here about spirit or soul. Mind is something different. It's the everyday place we occupy each and every day. It's what we know: a symbolic world, which, though seemingly derived from a biological brain, is *not* biological itself. Confusing, I know, but it's important for you to understand this distinction when you are looking for a psychiatrist.

You want a psychiatrist who appreciates the mind as the place where we live our lives *narratively*, as a unique, evolving story—a world distinctly unlike the deterministic workings of brain/body; a world where meaning and choice reside; one that defies biological explanation. Imaginative mind and biological brain—they are as different as hardware and software. Just as we can't decipher a software program from its computer hardware, we can't understand the world of mind by tallying up neurons and neurotransmitters. The words I write at this moment on a word processor emerge from a binary series of numbers. The words make narrative sense; the ones and zeros, digital sense. They are not the same, and they can't be meaningfully explained in similar terms.

TWO WORLDS, TWO LANGUAGES

I know I risk being overly dense here; but this is an important concept. You don't want all your time taken up by a psychiatrist who gives no consideration to mind problems you face in your day-to-day life. This is what will happen if your psychiatrist sees all things biological. Let me try to address the difference between mind and brain in a slightly different way. Matters of brain/body lend themselves to a mechanical language best suited for describing pumps, hydraulics, neurotransmitters, receptors, and energy exchange, but when applied to the subjective world of mind, this language fails miserably. In contrast, mind language, while not nearly as good at delineating a broken bone or stomach ulcer, is much more useful capturing imagination, awareness, motivation, and beliefs; much more suited to describing the human condition with its joys, sorrows, dilemmas, paradoxes, and mystical experiences. Mind language reflects our experience of consciousness and willful living and allows us to frame human problems in ways that suggest non-biological remedies. With reference to painful emotions and moods such as depression, mind language helps us understand what might be going wrong in our lives and why it's happening. It facilitates the understanding of *unique* life stories, something brain/body language cannot do.

Consider a comparison of appendicitis and romantic love. Trying to explain an inflamed appendix in mind language—in terms of motivations, intentions, guilt, and anger—would be futile. Mind language isn't helpful dealing with temperature, white blood cell counts, and abdominal rebound tenderness. Similarly, biological language isn't well suited for conveying life stories unfolding in the world of mind. Brain/body language has no words helpful in clarifying the part a person plays in his or her own depression. When human feelings such as romantic love or guilt are reduced to neurotransmitter language, something essential is lost in translation. The fact that researchers scan the brain and see various parts light up with different emotions says nothing about the personal meaning of those emotions. Brain imaging cannot help with *personal* problems.

A psychiatrist must venture beyond chemical imbalance. This requires being fully conversant in mind language. Otherwise, he or she will be greatly disadvantaged trying to help you. You want a psychiatrist who understands and feels comfortable in the world of mind.

STRADDLING MIND AND BRAIN/BODY

Even though mind and brain/body are not the same, they strongly influence each other. An image may trigger an asthma attack; an imagined stress may cause a heart attack. The person seemingly made anxious by losing her job may discover later that the anxiety was the product of an overactive thyroid, not job loss. Unfortunately, the great promise of psychosomatic medicine has yet to be fully realized. Despite dramatic examples of mind/brain interaction such as stunted growth in children of dysfunctional families, psychologically induced immunological changes, and a host of medical conditions powerfully influenced by mind stress—the connections between mind and body remain only vaguely understood.

Psychiatry's great promise lies in straddling these separate but connected worlds. But, historically, psychiatrists have resisted this role, gravitating toward one or the other domain but not both. In the early nineteenth century a biological view proved useful in finding a successful treatment of mental derangement caused by syphilis and tuberculosis. But in time psychiatry's focus shifted to the mind, most notably in the form of Freudian psychology. By mid–twentieth century, with the waning of Freudian influence and after a brief flirtation with community mental health, psychiatry resumed its biological bias, this time emphasizing neurotransmitters, neuroreceptors, and "chemical imbalance." Leon Eisenberg, a Harvard psychiatrist, described psychiatry as "brainless" the first half of the twentieth century and "mindless" the second half. Along with this shift came a decline in psychiatrists' ability to deal with the human condition.

For some, the suggestion that psychiatrists embrace mind as well as brain/body will seem a preposterous idea, an absurd throwback. The way is clear, they say: better living through chemistry is psychiatry's future. This stance leaves clinical psychiatrists severely limited in what they can do for their patients and deprives modern medicine of a true psychosomatic discipline.

Among mental health professionals, psychiatrists are unique in their complete medical training. Increasingly, however, this distinction means little. After finishing medical school, most psychiatrists let their medical skills gradually lapse, even though for economic purposes they hold tight to the M.D. behind their names. One study showed fully a third of psychiatrists unable to perform a physical examination (Pomeroy et al. 2002). This decline starts with residency. General medicine concerns give way to a devouring preoccupation with psychodrugs. My view of psychiatry's proper place has the psychiatrist, first and foremost, a solid M.D. Don't settle for a psychiatrist who is no longer a competent physician. For what purpose? you might ask.

PSYCHOLOGICAL MASQUERADES

Medical problems often aggravate psychiatric symptoms without the awareness of patients or their psychiatrists. This is especially true of cardiovascular disease, diabetes, obstructive pulmonary disease, hepatitis, hypothyroidism, and fluid and electrolyte disorders (Sokal et al. 2004; Carney et al. 2006). Consider the symptom of depression. While this painful emotion typically arises from adverse life experiences, there are a variety of medical causes: stroke, diabetes, chronic obstructive pulmonary disease, AIDS, or other neurological diseases. Vascular depression (associated with MRI changes in the basal ganglia) accounts for roughly 50 percent of late-life depressions (Yohanes and Baldwin 2008). In coronary heart disease, there's a two-way interaction. Depression increases the risk of heart problems; and, in turn, heart problems make a person twice as likely to become depressed. This same relationship applies to diabetes (type II) and depression. Diabetes substantially increases the risk of depression, and being depressed leaves a patient more vulnerable to developing diabetes. The risk for diabetes rises by 50 percent when a person takes an antidepressant psychodrug (Pan et al. 2010).

To further complicate psychiatric diagnosis, some persons with depression also have cognitive problems such as memory loss and difficulty solving simple problems—symptoms suggestive of dementia. In fact many of these patients are misdiagnosed initially as suffering from Alzheimer's disease, only to experience complete cognitive recovery as their depression clears. Psychiatrists who remain competent physicians are best prepared to identify cases such as "pseudodementia" and to detect various medical conditions that mimic psychiatric disorders. Roughly 10 percent of "psychiatric" cases turn out to be psychological masquerades such as brain tumors presenting as depression, pneumonia as panic attacks, atypical seizures as psychosis, and a host of adverse medication reactions as various psychological and behavioral changes. And these are only a few of the myriad of masquerading conditions that psychiatrists should detect and treat or appropriately refer to other physicians (Taylor 2007; Koran et al. 1989).

Masquerades come in strange packages. I recall a middle-aged man, a university professor, who complained of debilitating panic attacks. The only good thing about these episodes was that they were limited to weekends, mainly Sunday mornings. One therapist told the man he probably was feeling anxious being away from his university work! As I delved deeper into his weekend routine, I discovered his beloved ritual of drinking coffee and reading the paper. When I say drinking coffee, I mean lots of coffee. On Sunday mornings with a copy of the *New York Times*, the man sometimes consumed eight to ten cups. When I suggested to him that his panic attacks might be the result of excessive caffeine consumption, he found this hard to believe but agreed to avoid coffee the following weekend. At our next session, the man reported no more panic attacks but was quick to conclude that probably it was just a coincidence. It took three more weekends with no further panic attacks to convince him otherwise. By this time he had also discovered that his older sister had suffered panic attacks years earlier from drinking too much coffee. In our java-laden society, caffeinism is a common problem with its increased anxiety, tremulousness, and sometimes even panic.

Given a rapidly aging population, cognitive decline is becoming more prevalent. Although this deficit does not progress invariably to full-blown dementia, any degree of cognitive impairment has serious consequences. Psychiatrists should be expert at assessing cognition and skilled at counseling patients on ways of minimizing and adapting to cognitive changes, mild to severe.

Adverse medication effects represent a major cause of cognitive decline, especially those related to psychodrugs. I remember an older woman, probably in her late seventies, I saw as an outpatient. Just before her appointment, the social worker pulled me aside to tell me that this charming lady had contracted dementia. A few minutes later she escorted a stooped and slightly disheveled person into my office. Tremulous and unsteady, the woman appeared frightened and confused. I inquired as to how she was doing. "Not so good," she whispered anxiously. Although she knew where she was, when I asked her the date, she was off by several years. I listed four items—a horse, a car, a lamp, and a table—for her to remember. When, a few minutes later, I asked her to recall them, she struggled to remember any. Dementia was a definite possibility, but upon glancing over her medications, I discovered the woman was on *seven* different psychodrugs, which I realized could be part of the problem. Her social worker and I discussed how her case manager was to help her taper off the psychiatric medications. Two weeks later when I saw her again, she was a changed woman. Meticulously dressed, regal appearing with her silver-gray hair, she entered my office, steady and confident. At one point she joked about having felt the "fog" lift. What appeared to be dementia turned out to be severe confusion from psychodrugs. Once the medications cleared her system, the woman was her normal self again.

If you start on a psychodrug, you want a psychiatrist who is quick to recognize side effects. Surprisingly, many psychiatrists are only vaguely familiar with the full spectrum of adverse effects. Also, other kinds of medication can cause similar effects. Earlier in my career, working as a psychiatric consultant to hospitalized medical and surgical patients, I became quite familiar with this problem. Typically, I would be called to see a patient who was described as "acting crazy" and thought to be a candidate for transfer to the psychiatric service. In many cases a quick review of the troubled patient's medications (sometimes, quite extensive) provided the answer to the sudden change in behavior. The solution was simply to stop the offending medication. In an era when problematic drug concoctions frequently arise from patients having multiple doctors, medication-induced behavioral changes are on the rise. With a rapidly aging population that, on average, takes a staggering number of medications, we stand on the brink of a toxicity epidemic. It's valuable to have a psychiatrist exquisitely sensitive to this potential problem.

Overall, good medical care enhances psychiatric care.

In one study a designated group of mental health patients received extra medical oversight. Special case managers facilitated access to appropriate medical care. After twelve months, the oversight group experienced superior *psychiatric* improvement: 8 percent versus a decline of 1.1 percent in routine care patients (Druss et al. 2010). Persons seeking psychiatric help commonly suffer from complicating medical conditions. Even so, a national survey of 181 community mental health centers found only a third included medical services and only half made medical referrals (Druss et al. 2008).

TAKING ON ADDICTIONS

Traditionally, psychiatrists have resisted treating addictions. But this long-standing practice of separating addiction from other psychiatric problems makes no clinical sense. Why should psychiatrists work with other kinds of obsessive/compulsive problems and avoid compulsive substance use? Addictions to alcohol, street drugs, and prescription drugs predictably destroy lives, exacerbate psychiatric symptoms, and sometimes cause new ones. They are also associated with a host of complicating medical problems. In terms of total human costs, no other psychiatric condition causes a greater toll. Given that drug and alcohol problems are much more common among psychiatric patients than the general population, in a break with the past, psychiatrists should be fully engaged in both identifying and treating addictions.

Most addicted persons I've known have excelled at hiding their problem, at least for a while. They lie to others and they lie to themselves. Psychiatrists should be particularly sensitive to the possibility of addiction confusing the psychiatric picture and often causing serious medical complications. As for addictive behavior itself, there are no easy answers and no one best treatment. What works for one person fails for another. For some patients construing the addictive behavior as a "medical disease" is helpful; for others, this explanation falls flat. For some, self-help groups are essential; for others, they don't work. Psychiatrist should be familiar with various approaches including motivational counseling, addiction groups, and medications such as naloxone, buprenorphine, nicotine replacement, and bupropion, and they should be alert to the possible need for residential care and work/treatment programs as a way of helping a patient make the long journey back.

Whatever approach a psychiatrist takes with addictions, persistence is key. Persons who finally "kick the habit," often, have had repeated failures. Each failure should be seen as a building block to ultimate success. Along the way, there will be a fine line between encouraging, supporting, treating, and enabling. The treatment challenges of addiction equal those of severe mental disability, but as it currently stands too often addiction is neglected. It's much too serious a problem for psychiatry to remain on the sideline.

Among addictions, I include smoking. A Canadian study found 40–80 percent of psychiatric patients—depending on their particular problem—smoked daily compared with 20 percent of the general public (Morisano et al. 2009). As addictions go, smoking is number one with respect to adverse health consequences. Some psychiatrists are reluctant to confront smoking out of concern that this may aggravate a patient's psychiatric problems. But a review of studies over the past fifteen years failed to find convincing evidence for this assumption. To the contrary depression declined once substance abuse was controlled (Kelly 2009). If excessive use of drugs or alcohol contributes to your problems, choose a psychiatrist experienced in dealing with addictions. Many are not.

Unfortunately, many psychiatrists are also woefully uninformed about hormones and their influence on behavior. It's my experience that few are very knowledgeable about the hormonal underpinnings of psychiatric symptoms or about the therapeutic use of hormone replacement for psychiatric symptoms. The role of replacement hormones in postmenopausal women has become hopelessly confused by a myriad of conflicting reports, leaving many women to fend for themselves. There is good evidence that supplemental hormones and hormone precursors help ameliorate psychiatric symptoms and provide some women *and* men a significantly better quality of life. In a small study of twenty-two women with major

depression, half received the hormone precursor dehydroepiandrosterone (DHEA) and half, placebo. At the end of six weeks,
five of the eleven women on DHEA (maximum of 90 mg daily)
showed 50 percent or less depression as compared with the
women on placebo, *none* of whom showed such improvement
(Wolkowitz et al. 1999). A second study of DHEA supplementation focused on midlife-onset depression. Of twenty-six patients
taking DHEA, twenty-three experienced at least 50 percent
improvement as compared with thirteen of twenty-six on placebo (Schmidt et al. 2005).

Severe premenstrual syndrome—a cyclical hormonal
condition—can be mistaken for bipolar disorder and treated
ineffectively with antidepressants and mood stabilizers as
opposed to targeting the real problem: hormone imbalance.
There are reports of long-standing "bipolar depression" *disap-
pearing* with the "suppression of ovarian cycles" (Studd 2012).
Finally, the proper role of hormone replacement in postmenopausal depression remains a seriously neglected topic in psychiatry. If you develop this problem in midlife, make certain
your psychiatrist evaluates your hormone levels and considers
hormone replacement as frontline treatment if there are no
contraindications.

Solid medical grounding serves psychiatrists well as they
treat mental and emotional problems related to pregnancy, the
postpartum period, and menopause. These are the psychiatrists
best positioned to use findings such as the recent report that,
midpregnancy, placental corticotrophin-releasing hormone
may predict postpartum depression (Yim et al. 2009). You definitely want a psychiatrist who understands the importance of
hormonal balance for your mental and emotional life.

RECLAIMING MEDICAL CREDENTIALS

Absent medical skills, psychiatrists are indistinguishable from other mental health professionals. Already, nonmedical professionals (nurse practitioners, physician assistants, and psychologists, in some states) can prescribe psychodrugs. But full medical training potentially gives psychiatrists a unique advantage dealing with mind/body issues. Up until a few decades ago, psychiatrists dominated psychosomatic medicine. No longer. Psychiatrists should reassert this dominance. They should be knowledgeable consultants on medical problems unduly influenced by psychological factors: conditions such as fibromyalgia, irritable bowel syndrome, chronic fatigue, eating disorders, chronic pain syndromes, and tension headaches. These mystifying disorders deserve more medically informed psychiatric attention. A six-year study of 2,400 middle-aged men found those who exhibited the greatest sense of "hopelessness" at greatest risk of dying early from heart disease and cancer (Everson et al. 1996). You want a psychiatrist who truly understands the powerful interaction of mind and body and takes both into account as he or she works with you.

In the psychosomatic category I would include chronic pain. This is an area where few psychiatrists venture. Given the medical-legal risks associated with prescribing narcotics and other painkillers, I understand the hesitation. Still, psychiatry is a field desperate for new roles that more fully integrate mind and brain/body insights, and chronic pain merits special attention.

Years ago George Engel, distinguished dean of psychosomatic medicine, famously castigated general medicine for its narrow "biomedical model" of disease. In an article titled "The Need for a New Medical Model: A Challenge for Biomedicine," he commented: "The dominant model of disease today is bio-medical, and it leaves no room within its framework for the social, psychological, and behavioral dimensions of illness" (Engel 1977). If Engel were still alive, I suspect he would be aghast at how much his critique applies to *psychiatrists*.

In summary, select a psychiatrist who remains a competent physician; one who truly understands how medical problems and medications complicate psychiatric problems, how what appears "psychiatric" may be a manifestation of medical disease, and how the mind and body powerfully affect each other. Still, for your psychiatrist to be a competent physician is not enough. He or she must also embrace the world of mind. It's this dual competency that makes the *complete* psychiatrist.

In the next chapter I begin a discussion of mind work.

CHAPTER SIX

Mind Work I

Stories Gone Wrong and How to Fix Them

- Find a psychiatrist comfortable working in the world of mind.

- Choose one who will help you understand your personal style.

- Look for humility in a psychiatrist; shun arrogance.

- Reject the one who shows no interest in your personal story.

- Look for a personable, creative, and confident psychiatrist who inspires your trust.

Early in his career, Sigmund Freud imagined a "scientific psychology." He aspired to reveal the mind as an exact parallel to the brain. This was an early version of what later became the mantra of biological psychiatry: "a twisted molecule behind every twisted thought." But after making little headway, Freud gave up in frustration. More than a century later, no one else has

made much progress either. Still, there remain those neuroscientists (and many psychiatrists) who insist that eventually mind
will be fully translated into brain, after which all quaint psychological descriptions will seem nothing more than humorous
reminders of our troglodytic past. Regardless, for the moment
we go on living our lives in a subjective world of mind. We
don't experience our daily lives as a matter of brain mechanics.
For this reason, in many gatherings of well-educated people,
a recently trained psychiatrist might well have the least cogent
things to say about why people behave, think, and feel the way
they do. Why? Because by viewing human behavior, thoughts,
and feelings primarily through a chemical lens, psychiatrists
tend to neglect human experience as it's lived.

In its dismissal of mind, psychiatry resembles behavioral psychology of the past century. The behaviorists burst onto the scene
claiming the mind was irrelevant; after all, it was only imaginary.
What mattered was behavior, something you could observe and
measure. Troubled behavior was a matter of misaligned con-
tingencies and misplaced rewards. Change was straightforward:
modify what was rewarded and what was punished and, presto,
the aberrant behavior would disappear and with it all the twisted
thoughts and emotions. But behavior therapy quickly flamed out
as it proved no match for complicated human dilemmas. When a
psychiatrist construes all psychiatric problems as chemical imbalance, he or she makes the same mistake behaviorists did earlier
when they failed to acknowledge the importance of the mind.

STORIES WE LIVE BY

From genes, memories, and experience, the mind—one of life's
great mysteries—emerges. Contrary to what many detractors

claim, the mind is not imaginary. It is a symbolic world anchored by a personal narrative in which each of us is the central character in his or her story. It could hardly be more real; after all, the mind is where human experience occurs.

The mind has its own set of rules, distinctly different from those of the brain/body. Unlike medical diseases, mind problems are symbolic matters, more akin to conflicts in novels and plays than to electrochemical malfunctions. The great Russian writer Joseph Conrad once observed: "Everything begins with a story." There's a simple reason for this: story serves as the mind's main currency. That's why, in order to be of optimal help to their patients, psychiatrists must understand stories. "We are all tellers of tales," writes Dr. Dan McAdams, author of *The Stories We Live By*. "We each seek to provide our scattered and often confusing experiences with a sense of coherence by arranging the episodes of our lives into stories. This is not the stuff of delusion or self-deception. We are not telling ourselves lies. Rather, through our personal stories myths, each of us discovers what is true and what is meaningful in life" (McAdams 1993). Daniel Taylor in *The Healing Power of Stories* says it this way: "Broken stories can be healed. . . . We are free to change the stories by which we live" (Taylor 1966).

Characteristically, stories center on a protagonist—each of us—who, in trying to live a meaningful life, inevitably confronts obstacles. These obstacles may be experienced as a disparity between self-image and reality, as interpersonal struggles for intimacy, inclusion, and control, or as life stressors in the form of financial, academic, occupational, or cultural challenges. At the heart of all these problems is a gap between what we want or need and what we have. How we manage these challenges determines how well we value ourselves. When the gap between what we face and what we can handle becomes too great, we feel overwhelmed, our self-confidence and sense of hope threatened. But when challenges are handled successfully, we move ahead feeling more confident and optimistic.

Whoever we are—whatever diagnoses we have or don't have—on occasion our stories go off track: they take unexpected turns for the worse, sometimes because of what we've done and, at other times, simply because bad things happen. On these occasions we sometimes need help, at least temporarily, in the way of supportive understanding, feedback, guidance, and assistance in better understanding our personal story. At the same time we need to learn from our experiences so as to reduce the chances as much as possible of having similar problems in the future.

In your search for a psychiatrist beware of how psychiatry as a discipline has lost touch with story. With cursory attention to personal story, too many psychiatrists rush through the machinations of a "mental status examination" with a narrow focus on diagnosis and the psychodrugs. Time is short; more patients are coming. Insurers want less talk and more medication. Managed care, the same. Whatever your particular individual story, when a psychiatrist finishes "working you up," too often, it has been reduced to a tale of bad chemistry. If you are not careful in your selection, more likely than not your psychiatrist will have little understanding of what is upsetting your life and what might be done other than taking pills.

Even patients for whom psychodrugs are essential have personal problems that defy simplistic chemical explanations. Paul McHugh, professor of psychiatry emeritus at Johns Hopkins and author of *The Mind Has Mountains*, puts story at the heart of all mind work: "all psychotherapists eventually compose with the patient's cooperation some kind of story—a chronicle that reveals how psychological symptoms arise when such motivations as hopes, commitments, preferences, and fears collide with reality" (McHugh 2006). The psychiatrist and anthropologist Arthur Kleinman makes a similar point: "The psychiatrist's work," he insists, "is chiefly about people's life stories. It is about aspirations and defeats, about passions and tragedies" (Kleinman 1988).

Harvey Chochinov, a Canadian psychiatrist, pioneered a narrative approach to dying he called *Dignity Therapy*. The basic idea is to help patients compose a written record of their lives that will live on after they die, something loved ones can touch and read for its memories and insights. Chochinov recounts how at the end of therapy the stories people tell about themselves differ greatly from earlier versions. He views this as an expression of the universal, unending search for meaning (Chochinov et al. 2005). It also reminds us that our personal stories are constantly being revised as we struggle to put together a meaningful life.

Choose a *mindful* psychiatrist. One who pays attention to your personal story. A failure to listen to *individual* stories proved the ultimate downfall of psychoanalysis. Too quickly all observations were reduced to stock Freudian conflicts and treated with standard psychoanalytic techniques. If the patient's problems failed to fit the psychoanalytic worldview, too bad; psychoanalysis was correct. The patient's unique story became obscured in the strained convolutions of psychoanalytic dogma. Too often the same seems true of other "franchise" therapies such as cognitive behavioral therapy (CBT), interpersonal therapy (IPT), and dialectic behavior therapy (DBT). These off-the-shelf, one-size-fits-all therapies push a certain worldview and standard treatment strategy that discourages a more nuanced understanding of you.

You want a psychiatrist who has mastered a variety of mind tools from which he or she can selectively draw and apply to you and your particular situation. At its best, mind work is a highly individualized endeavor, custom designed to fit a particular consumer's problems. Don't settle for less.

UNDERSTANDING PERSONALITY

Who you are is central to *your* story. Each of us has a distinct personality, reflecting enduring styles of feeling, thinking, and behaving. Interwoven into this personality are dominant values, fears, and desires. Apart from labeling a few difficult types, most psychiatrists pay little attention to personality. This is a mistake. We can't very well understand patients' stories without knowing *who* they are. This requires that we look beyond what is covered in a standard psychiatric workup.

Personalities emerge out of early traits (temperament) present at birth (Thomas and Birch 1970; Kagan and Snidman 2004). We enter the world with varying degrees of reactivity, impulsiveness, adaptability, persistence, distractibility, relatedness, and so forth. As we grow, life situations and personal relationships elaborate these traits into more complete personalities crucial to how we go about adapting to life's demands. An understanding of our personalities—strengths and weaknesses—is a special kind of knowledge that helps us adapt to life's demands and relate more satisfactorily to other people.

Insist that your psychiatrist, among other things, help you better understand your own personality. This is invaluable information. Sometimes this is pursued as a clinical exploration, but there are a variety of personality tests your psychiatrist can utilize. Some of the best known are based on the five-factor model of core personality traits: openness (curious/cautious), conscientiousness (self-disciplined/ spontaneous), extroversion (outgoing/withdrawn), agreeableness (cooperative/antagonistic), and neuroticism (insecure/ confident). This perspective maintains that personalities are a blend of these five traits. The Sixteen Personality Factor Questionnaire, otherwise known as the 16-PF, claims to use a refinement of the five-factor model. As its name implies, it yields sixteen personality types (Cattell 1989), each with its own characteristic ways of thinking, perceiving, feeling, and behaving.

In their book *Personality Self-Portrait*, John Oldham and Lois Morris offer another view of personality as they describe thirteen dimensions—conscientious, self-confident, dramatic, vigilant, mercurial, devoted, solitary, leisurely, sensitive, idiosyncratic, adventurous, self-sacrificing, and aggressive—that blend together in various combinations (Oldham and Morris 1990). The Enneagram provides yet another way of understanding personality. Based on various mixes of three basic dimensions— feeling, thinking, and instinctive—nine personality styles are identified such as helper, achiever, and challenger (Riso and Hudson 1999).

But the most widely used personality test is the Myers-Briggs Type Indicator. Inspired by Jungian psychology, the test identifies four major dichotomies of personal style: (1) extroversion/ introversion: the way a person gets energized and relates to others, (2) sensing/intuiting: how a person takes in information, (3) thinking/feeling: the dominant basis for making decisions, and (4) judging/perceiving: the speed and permanence of decision making. Typically, each of us leans more toward one or the other of these four dichotomies. Overall scores indicate one of sixteen personality types (Meyers and Meyers 1980).

Keep in mind, as with psychiatric diagnoses, personality typing, if overemphasized, can be misleading. At best it provides a rough guide, but one that can be invaluable in helping you better understand conflicts in your life story.

Personality assessment's greatest value comes from the insights you derive about your particular personal style. What initial impressions do you make? What are your main strengths and weaknesses? What things in life are most important to you? What are your passions? Your values? What are your greatest pleasures? Your strongest motivators? Does your personality play a major role in repetitive patterns of problematic behavior? With a deeper understanding of your personality, you and your psychiatrist are better prepared to explore your personal story and how it may have gotten off track.

You may find it surprising when I say it's also important you pay attention to your *psychiatrist's* personality. To be sure you want a technically competent psychiatrist, but you also want a psychiatrist who listens and gets to know you and your special story. Nowhere else in medicine is a doctor's personality and how it meshes with your own so critical. Research shows that psychotherapy depends more on the therapist's personality (and the therapeutic relationship) than on any particular therapeutic approach. Personality traits that strongly correlate with better outcomes include: genuine concern, empathy, and supportive respect (Patterson 1984). Additionally, Jerome Frank's exhaustive review of psychotherapy suggests that the confidence a psychiatrist (or any other therapist) projects—more than any specific approach he or she uses—signals the best chance of success (Frank and Frank 1991). In short, much of mind work depends more on who the therapist is and on how he or she relates to you than on any special technique. You want a psychiatrist who is personable, respectful, and competent enough to earn your trust.

Over my career, I have known psychiatrists who were exceptionally good with patients. I have also known psychiatrists for whom patients appeared to be little more than a necessary inconvenience. Their oversize egos, self-absorption, and arrogance seemed destined to be major impediments to good therapy. If any healing took place, I figured it was in spite of their personalities. There was a time when personal psychotherapy was a requisite of psychiatric training, a way for a young psychiatrist to better know himself, particularly his or her rough edges. But with psychiatry's retreat from the world of mind, this expectation has disappeared. This is unfortunate given that personality awareness is such an essential element of therapy.

As a consumer, trust your instincts. If you come across a psychiatrist with whom you feel uncomfortable much of the time, find someone else. But I hasten to add, guard against rejecting a psychiatrist simply because the going gets difficult. Mind work, particularly when you are forced to see the part you play in a problem you have attributed to someone else, can be emotionally painful. Sometimes it is easier to blame the psychiatrist than to admit one's own responsibility. There is a difference between sticking with a psychiatrist who accurately confronts you about problematic behavior and one who is aloof, dogmatic, and uninterested in anything more than a diagnosis.

In order to understand your story your psychiatrist must listen—*really listen*. I'm talking about listening that concentrates more on your story than on the answers to traditional psychiatric interview questions. Listening that allows for comments from you about the doctor-patient relationship. Listening that convinces you of his or her genuine concern and respect. Such listening is the best guarantee that your psychiatrist experiences you as a unique person and will provide authentic, empathetic treatment.

In his book *A Whole New Mind*, Daniel Pink explains how good listening underlies empathy. "Empathy is the ability to imagine yourself in someone else's position and to intuit what that person is feeling. It is the ability to stand in others' shoes, to see with their eyes, and to feel with their hearts." Empathy, he continues, is like "climbing into another's mind to experience the world from that person's perspective" (Pink 2005). If you mistakenly choose a psychiatrist who doesn't listen, chances are you won't find him very empathetic. My advice is to move on.

MIND WORK CONCEPTS

More art form than science, mind work resists production-line approaches. While stories are universal, each person's story is unique. This is why mind work defies standard approaches. Ultimately, the best psychotherapy resembles the best craftsman tradition, unbound by hard-and-fast rules. Even so, a variety of strategies employed by an artful psychiatrist or therapist can be extremely helpful. What follows is a discussion of concepts, tools, and techniques I have found particularly useful. I start with concepts.

Emotions are flares from the mind. Sometimes they appear on the surface but not always. Sometimes they remain suppressed, detectable only as subtle cues easily missed unless a psychiatrist pays close attention. The psychological pain that psychiatric patients commonly experience often goes unexpressed. Stuffing our feelings is a common human foible. This is why psychiatrists must be exquisitely attuned to emotions. They often provide valuable clues to a story reluctantly told. One of my former psychiatry professors, Fred Melges, described emotions as expressions of self-appraisal, internal signals of how we perceive our lives are going. When things are working well, we feel up; when they turn sour, we feel anxious, depressed, or angry, sometimes even confused, suspicious, or hopeless. Negative emotions reflect a widening gap—actual or anticipated—between what a person has and what he or she wants; between what a person aspires to be and his or her self-image. This view of emotions as informative messages clashes with the prevailing idea that negative emotions *are* the problem. Get rid of the bad emotions, solve the problem. This perspective ignores the *meaning* behind emotional reactions.

Daniel Siegal, UCLA clinical professor of psychiatry and author of *Mindsight*, describes a "seventh sense." "It lets us 'name and tame' the emotions we are experiencing," he says, "rather than be overwhelmed. A good psychiatrist makes use of this seventh sense to help you get in touch with your emotions and make better use of them." Siegal illustrates the value of working with emotions by distinguishing between *being* sad and *feeling* sad. The first interpretation—being sad—leaves a person in a passive position, unable to do anything about the way he or she is. The second perspective—feeling sad—encourages a more active response. It's easier to change the way you feel than to change the way you are. Sensing an emotion as a transitory feeling opens up the possibility of change and mastery as opposed to feeling stuck in a hopeless situation (Siegal 2010).

Emotions reflect a subtle balance. The imaginative social psychologist, Leon Festinger showed how emotions, thoughts, and behavior are aligned. When these three aspects of our lives are out of sync, psychological tension (*dissonance*) develops. Dissonance, in turn, spurs compensatory changes in our emotions, beliefs, and behavior so as to bring them back into alignment (Festinger 1957). A shift in any of these dimensions induces "sympathetic" alterations in the others.

This "dissonance" principle can sometimes be put to good use by a psychiatrist trying to help a reluctant patient change a troubling behavior. Perhaps the patient has taken a new job and now has to start her day much earlier than usual. Being a "late" sleeper, our patient quickly finds herself in hot water after being late several times. Defeated, she tells her psychiatrist she sees no way out. She can't make herself get up. She will just have to look for another job. But what if, with her psychiatrist's encouragement, she makes a list of good things that will come from changing her sleep habits. When she goes home, she presents the list to her husband and kids, as her psychiatrist has insisted. Now she's *on record* advocating the advantages of early rising. She feels a heightened obligation. When she thinks about not following through, she gets a little anxious. It's enough to get her started, and even though initially she feels half asleep upon awakening, she rises early and goes to work, telling herself it won't last but persisting because *she said she would.* Her verbalized commitment keeps her at the task long enough for her to finally embrace this new behavior with praise from her family and respect from the people at work.

Years ago, when I was a first-year psychiatric resident at Stanford, Professor Irvin Yalom (an up-and-coming authority on group therapy) took a sabbatical. Before he left, our residency group asked if we could undertake a group therapy research project while he was away. With Yalom's blessing, we designed a study to compare the efficacy of several different group approaches. For patients to be accepted into one of our groups, they had to fill out lengthy assessments and personality tests. It was an arduous process and took hours to complete.

At the conclusion of the study, much to our dismay, we failed to turn up a superior approach. All the groups fared about the same. Even so, we made a fascinating discovery. One of the problems Yalom had struggled with was dropouts. Commonly, half of his group participants stopped attending within a few weeks. In contrast, the groups we put together had few dropouts. Eventually, we concluded that unwittingly we had created dissonance in our participants by subjecting them to such rigorous (and in retrospect probably unreasonable) entry requirements. Any thought of dropping out was countered by the distasteful memory of excessive time and effort spent getting accepted. We assumed this translated into extra commitment. After putting up with all the admission hurdles, the participants weren't about to quit. Dissonance at work! Years later I came across work by Elliot Aronson and Judson Mills in an article titled "The Effect of Severity of Initiation on Liking for a Group," supportive of this dissonance explanation (Aronson and Mills 1959).

In his book *A Theory of Personality: The Psychology of Personal Constructs*, Dr. George Kelly outlines a particularly creative use of dissonance which he calls *fixed role therapy* (Kelly 1963). Kelly describes a young woman who had become hopelessly dissatisfied with her life. With encouragement, she agreed to work on "imaging" the kind of person she wanted to be. Together, Kelly and the patient worked out detailed changes in dress, public presentation, socializing, entertaining, relationships, vacationing, and free time. In addition they outlined specific plans for making new friends, finding a different job, and pursuing new avenues of personal development. As homework the patient filled in the details until she felt comfortable with how they fit together as a whole. Once this "new" person was fully created, like an actress assuming a new character, the patient assumed the role in her everyday life. Kelly describes how she gradually progressed from feeling like she was acting to eventually living this new identity. This novel approach to character change makes full use of the dissonance principle. A voluntary change in behavior and appearance—even when assumed as a "role"—eventually causes a compensatory shift in attitude and self-image. Over the years, I have found variations on this idea invaluable in helping patients change.

Psychotherapy researcher Jerome Frank saw a different kind of dissonance in his depressed patients. He characterized their central emotion as *demoralization*, explaining that their life stories run amuck until they become exhausted, feeling trapped and hopeless. With their future seemingly nothing but a black hole in contrast to their aspirations, they give up. Frank maintained that simple acts of understanding and encouragement, along with help replacing negative, energy-draining assumptions with more realistic ones, was restorative (Frank and Frank 1991). He believed that a major contributor to demoralization was the "inability to make sense of what they were experiencing," which he likened to an incoherent story plot. This is why he urged therapists to collaborate with their patients in fashioning a different story, one more helpful explaining what had happened as well as suggesting solutions to what in the patient's mind had become insurmountable.

I've found *stress/distress* yet another useful mind work concept.

Each of us meets life's challenges with varying degrees of resiliency. For some, even modest challenges raise the terror of failure, while for others the most daunting threats are handled with cool confidence. Still, each person has a limit beyond which challenge becomes overwhelming. Within a person's limits, confronting and overcoming difficulties enhances self-esteem and self-assurance. But when challenges exceed our capacity, stress morphs into *distress* and gives rise to symptoms of anxiety, depression, irritability, faltering self-confidence, and learned helplessness (Seligman 1975).

The stress concept bridges mind and brain/body. Physiologically, mental stress is associated with the brain/body response to perceptions of a threat. Hearing a large animal coming toward you from the bushes nearby, for example, will cause a spike in your body's emergency-response steroid hormones (glucocorticoids). When the threat passes, these hormones dissipate. But in the modern world, many dangers of earlier human existence have given way to *symbolic* threats, which have a nasty habit of persisting. Unlike ancient threats that erupted out of the dark and were quickly resolved one way or the other, these symbolic dangers—often unresolved for extended periods—translate into distress and persistent elevations of stress hormones. In *Why Zebras Don't Get Ulcers*, Robert Sapolsky likens physiological distress to the experience of salmon swimming upstream against all obstacles back to their place of birth. At the conclusion of this harrowing ordeal, once these noble fish finally spawn, they physically deteriorate and quickly die, presumably the result of prolonged exposure to stress hormones (Sapolsky 2004). Human distress similarly takes its toll on brain/body as reflected in a variety of medical problems.

Across psychiatric diagnoses, patients confront stressors that threaten to overwhelm them. A psychiatrist can help in several ways. Some patients need a better understanding of how they contribute to such distress by "catastrophizing" relatively minor problems. Others can be logically walked through what they truly are facing and helped to clarify their options. (Persons disabled by stress symptoms sometimes need temporary stabilization with psychodrugs in order to better appraise what they are facing and what can be done about it.)

In my experience one of life's major stressors is the failure to accept certain inevitabilities. The "Serenity Prayer," attributed to the American theologian Reinhold Niebuhr, captures the idea when it distinguishes between what we can and cannot change and emphasizes the importance of understanding and accepting the difference. In his book *The Five Things We Cannot Change* David Richo summarizes life's unchangeable facts: (1) Regardless of what you want, life invariably changes and ends. (2) Despite the best of plans, things don't always work out. (3) At best, fairness occurs inconsistently. (4) Suffering cannot be avoided. (5) And people, even those you love, are not always loving in return (Richo 2006). For many patients part of the work that needs to be done involves facing up to life's inevitables, letting go, and moving on with renewed passion.

MIND WORK TOOLS

In the mid-1960s Herbert Benson, a Harvard cardiologist, conducted a long overdue, in-depth study of *meditation* (Wallace and Benson 1972). Based on this work, he went on to describe what he called "the relaxation response" (Benson and Klipper 2000). The beauty of this technique resides in its simplicity. There are only three elements: (1) a relaxed setting and (2) slow, deep breathing associated with a focusing word, phrase, or image, (3) performed for ten to twenty minutes once or twice daily. For many psychiatric patients, the relaxation response can be a valuable tool—one that can help a person modulate distress and one that all psychiatrists should be prepared to teach. When properly taught, self-induced relaxation provides relief for many persons suffering from anxiety, depression, drug abuse, and medical conditions such as high blood pressure, tension headaches, and fibromyalgia (Schneider et al. 2005; Kaplan et al. 1993; Kabat-Zinn et al. 1992). The fact that this procedure can be learned and self-administered promotes a sense of self-mastery and self-control. Benson's relaxation response provides an experience in mindfulness—a method of quieting the mind, calming excessive emotion, and sharpening one's focus. Regardless of a patient's diagnosis, increased mindfulness is a valuable asset.

Sometimes a person can minimize the impact of stress by changing his or her perspective, a tactic called *reframing*. A residency colleague of mine, Dr. Peter Bourne, spent time in Vietnam studying helicopter pilots. Flying a helicopter in this war zone was incredibly dangerous. Each time these men went up they stood a good possibility of being killed. So it was unexpected when Bourne found these men had low levels of stress steroids. This finding remained a mystery until Borne clarified some of the mental defenses these pilots were using. They seemed to control their stress by altering their perspectives. Sometimes the maneuver was little more than a self-deception. A pilot might look at the

date and based on something out of his past convince himself
it was his lucky day; or reason to himself that since a helicopter
had gone down the prior day, it was unlikely to happen two days
in a row. These men were modulating their stress reactions by
mentally *reframing* their situation so that they achieved a valuable
calmness without altering their performance alertness.

To help you reframe a situation, a psychiatrist must first
understand what you are facing and your view of it. Only then
can he or she assess the accuracy of your perception and whether
or not it seems amenable to reframing. Is the threat you are feeling overestimated? Are there alternative ways of understanding
the problem that make it less stressful psychologically and easier
to solve? Are there options you have not thought of or, perhaps,
have been unwilling to consider?

Many patients describe situations where they feel "stuck"—
trapped, seemingly with no way out. But these "impossible" situations often turn out otherwise if a patient can be persuaded
to think more creatively. Viewing a problem differently may be
all it takes to identify previously "invisible" solutions. Consider,
for example, a man involved in a troubled intimate relationship.
He no longer finds life with his partner satisfying. There is no
support, no fun, no passion, and they have many arguments.
The psychological pain has become almost unbearable; still, he
remains paralyzed in indecision. If he stays, nothing changes. If
he leaves, he feels no one else will want him. His psychiatrist,
sensing he is stuck, encourages the man to try and see things
from his partner's perspective. What is the situation like for her?
How would she describe their relationship? What would she say
are the major problems? What would she list as good aspects of
their relationship? What would she ask him to change? What
would he be willing to change? Putting ourselves in another

person's shoes (often devilishly difficult without help from someone else) constitutes a form of reframing that may serve to loosen an entrenched, self-defeating position. Sometimes a simple question—What if?—can be an effective perspective-changing device. What if you do walk out, what then? What if you stay and change the relationship? What if both of you change a little; how would things be different? Reframing can be an invaluable aid to someone stuck and miserable, but unable to change.

Years ago I read a fable that well illustrates the power of reframing. The story pits a beautiful maiden against a powerful tyrant. After the young woman refuses his advances several times, the tyrant finally corners her. With a fake smile, he tells her how he has given the matter much thought and has decided to let fate decide if they are meant for each other. As a crowd gathers, the tyrant explains in a loud voice so everyone can hear how he will place two stones—one white, one black—in a small velvet bag. The woman, he says, will then reach inside and draw out one of the stones. If she chooses black, she becomes his wife; but, if she chooses white, she is free to pursue her own way. Having set the stage, the man walks a short way down the path and, with his back turned to the crowd, picks up two black stones and puts them in the bag. Anxious and confused, the young woman has already surmised that this man will leave nothing to chance. Without seeing him do it, she knows somehow he will make certain that no matter which stone she chooses, he will have his way. And then it comes to her: there is no white stone. In that moment, her situation seems hopeless. But just as she reaches into the bag, an answer comes to her. She clutches one of the stones and then, before anyone can see, "accidentally" drops it among the rocks on the path. "What are you doing, woman!" the tyrant bellows, but the woman remains calm, now in complete control. She raises her hand and reassures the people gathered around. "No problem," she says. "We will know the color of the stone I chose from the color of the remaining one." With that she pulls out the other black stone and holds it high. "See, I chose the white one first," she asserts with a smile. The crowd applauds, and the tyrant, completely deflated, walks away. By simply reframing her situation, the woman turned defeat into victory.

Another variation of reframing involves encouraging patients to try something they fear. *Paradoxing*, as it's been called, often provides relief for patients overwhelmed by anxiety arising from the fear of failure (Haley 1990). The more they fail, the more anxious they become; the more anxious they become, the more they fail. Certain instances of male impotence fall into this category. The man is made so anxious by the thought of not having an erection that he becomes unable to perform sexually, which only serves to make him more anxious. This kind of problem—and others like it—sometimes resolves itself if the performance anxiety can be reduced. So, how does a psychiatrist (or therapist) help make this happen? One approach involves instructing the patient to fail! Although encouraging the person to touch and caress his partner, the psychiatrist tells him that under no circumstance is he to allow himself to have an erection. It's like giving the person a free pass. The thing he's come to fear is no longer an issue. The pressure is off. He's been instructed *not* to become erect. In this fail-safe context, it is not unusual for a man to overcome his problem by "failing" this assignment. Such "reverse psychology" often proves useful in a

variety of situations where the common denominator is performance anxiety. For the psychiatrist, the challenge is to recognize
this type of self-defeating behavior.

Another kind of dysfunctional behavior I commonly come
across is what I call *merry-go-rounds*. Time and time again some
persons repeat personal relationships that invariably end up prov-
ing unsatisfactory. Such persons need to understand why this
repetitive pattern—despite repeated failure and psychological
pain—persists. What is the invisible payoff that keeps it going?
Often when I first raise this question, the person resists, unwilling to even consider the possibility. Silly idea. Why would I do
this to myself? he or she may ask incredulously. Sometimes when
I point out the tremendous excitement involved in uproarious
endings, this is enough to get the person invested in searching
for the payoff in his or her life that perpetuates repeated self-
destructive behavior. Over my career, I have found merry-go-
rounds a frequent component of troubled life stories. Examples
include repeated disastrous love affairs, recurrent authority problems, and frequent quests that consistently prove unsatisfying.

Failure to understand the *periodic need for course correction*
underlies some of life's most common merry-go-rounds. Stay-
ing with stultifying jobs, destructive relationships, or misguided
pleasure pursuits seems easier than making a change. Often
with help perceiving the merry-go-round for what it is, a patient
gathers the courage to make a life-enhancing course correction.

Regardless of diagnosis, many persons struggle with personal relationships, often without understanding the problematic role they play. Sometimes I find it helpful to *provide a
framework for looking at relationships*. There are many possibilities. One I have often used is "transactional analysis," conceived
years ago by Eric Berne and popularized by Thomas Harris in

his clever book, *I'm Okay, You're Okay* (Berne 1964). This view of relationships explains how personal conflicts arise from crossed communication. Two persons, ostensibly equals, are unable to get along because unknowingly they treat each other as parent and child instead of two equal adults. This kind of crossed communication plays itself out as "games" that vary in intensity from disruptive to deadly. In order for these games to continue, both persons must persist in relating inappropriately while neither of them draws attention to what is going on. If one person stops, the game is over. Without understanding the *game nature* of troubled relationships, persons run the risk of continuing them for years, if not for life.

MIND WORK TECHNIQUES

With psychiatry so dominated by psychodrugs, today's psychiatry trainees receive little training in mind work techniques. By way of illustration, I'll mention three that I've found particularly helpful. The first is *deconditioning*. For reasons not well understood, some persons become extremely fearful of situations that most of us handle comfortably. They develop exaggerated fears of flying, public places, public speaking, elevators, heights, spiders, and so on. These irrational fears can be life disrupting. The good news is how often they can be overcome with reeducative deconditioning. This procedure exposes patients to a feared object or situation *virtually*, in a safe setting on repeated occasions. As a result of this "office" experience, in time, the person's irrational fear disappears. The technique is applied in the following way.

With the patient made to feel comfortable and relaxed, the psychiatrist (or therapist) has him or her imagine a series of scenes, starting with the least feared and advancing to the most feared. For example, someone terrified by the thought of riding an elevator might start with an image of walking through a park on the way to a tall building. As long as the patient remains relaxed, the images can be advanced: arriving at an intersection several blocks away, the tall building still at a distance but in full view, stopping at a newspaper stand at the building's entrance, entering the lobby, standing in front of the elevator with its doors closed, then open, stepping into the elevator, pushing a button, riding the elevator to the next floor and back down, and, finally, to the top. Having once completed the entire sequence successfully, the person often finds it possible to confront the real thing with much less trepidation.

For a psychiatrist, equally important to mastering the deconditioning technique is sensitivity to *unexpressed* irrational fears. Consider this hypothetical example. A man complains about his strained marriage. "Basic incompatibility," he says. His wife always wants to go out; he prefers to stay in. After several years, they both come to feel resentful, blaming each other. But with further elaboration, the man's psychiatrist—looking for other possible explanations—uncovers a problem the man has tried to keep secret, even from his wife. The thought of being in public places with strangers terrifies him. As a matter of pride, he has never told his wife. So, what appears on the surface to be an irreconcilable strain in the marriage turns out to be a problem of irrational fear, one that might well be amenable to deconditioning.

A second technique I find useful is *hypnosis*. Hypnosis has a long history shrouded in mystery and skepticism; it is often viewed more as a stage scam than a legitimate mind tool. When I was a psychiatric resident, Dr. Ernest Hilgard of

Stanford University, a noted hypnosis researcher, introduced me to its possibilities. He demythologized hypnosis, presenting it as more a special kind of relationship than a "clouding of the mind." The first professional paper I ever wrote was with my psychiatric colleague Dr. James Tenzel. As a way of testing the claim stated in various medical texts that human warts could be cured by suggestion, we designed a study involving persons who had warts on both hands. A few newspaper ads produced plenty of volunteers. We told them we would treat each of their hands with a different method. The first method consisted of hypnotizing the patient and then, while he or she remained in a light trance, making repeated suggestions that the warts on one hand would slowly disappear. Following this, we "treated" the patient's other hand for several minutes with a bright, purple-tinted light. (In actuality this was the placebo—the "power of suggestion"—we were comparing with hypnosis.) Even now I recall being impressed with the great variability in peoples' ability to be hypnotized. Many of our subjects were children who, on average, tend to be more hypnotizable than adults. But even among these young people, the capacity for "going under" proved highly variable (Tenzel and Taylor 1969). Hypnosis varies in effectiveness, working best with persons who are good subjects. There are easy ways of quickly determining hypnotic susceptibility: for example, getting positive responses to suggestions such as "While you are standing, close your eyes and imagine the wind blowing first from the front and then from the back," or "Focus on your hand; feel it growing lighter until it begins to slowly rise in the air." Hypnotizable persons readily follow such suggestions. Hypnosis can be a valuable aid in exploring personal conflicts and in helping with smoking cessation and weight loss. In addition to being an excellent tool for inducing the relaxation required for deconditioning, it can serve as a self-help technique for sleeplessness and for post-traumatic stress symptoms and anxiety attacks (Amen 2010.) I suspect few residency programs teach hypnosis any longer. Too bad. Despite its checkered history, the technique is one any resourceful psychiatrist can put to good use.

A third valuable technique is *negotiation*.

The best clinical psychiatrists are good negotiators. They accept the importance of being flexible in a highly intuitive and subjective discipline. They are willing to pay heed when you express your own ideas or question their assessments and recommendations. I recall a particular patient who, despite a long-lasting and severe depression, resisted the idea of taking medication. Afraid a psychodrug would make him sick, he remained adamantly opposed. When I felt we had reached a standoff, I took a different tack. I asked him if he would consider a compromise. He didn't answer right away but continued to listen. A good sign. I suggested how instead of his taking medication daily the way it was usually prescribed, perhaps he would consider taking it once a week in the beginning to be certain it wasn't too much. By the squint in his eye and raised eyebrow, I suspected he felt I was trying to pull a fast one, but he surprised me. "Once a week can't be enough," he insisted. "Tell you what: I'll take one every three days and come back in two weeks." At least the door was ajar. When the man returned, having now decided the medication was safe enough, he agreed to take it on a daily basis. This approach has the additional advantage of eliciting greater commitment from patients by their feeling they have participated in making the choice.

There is a counterpart to negotiation: *persuasion*. You want a psychiatrist who, when he thinks a course of action best for you, can be persuasive. Persons often need encouragement to put aside destructive patterns, to take medication, or to open themselves to new ways of experiencing. Motivating you to take a risk will be easier if your psychiatrist has a persuasive way.

TAKING THE TIME

Given the shrinking duration of psychiatric sessions, you might ask: how can there be enough time for matters of the mind? It's a reasonable question. Let me try to answer. For starters, no one has ever shown that duration of psychiatric treatment determines how helpful it is. Some of my most meaningful exchanges with patients are brief encounters: a simple observation, feedback on certain decisions or behavior, praise for a new insight or a more constructive action. With some patients I alternate the focus, concentrating on psychodrugs during one session and on real-life problems and mind work the next. Sometimes I do some of both during each session.

Exactly how your psychiatrist handles the time depends on you and your particular needs. During my years in private practice, I never understood managed care's insistence on two professionals instead of one in cases where combined psychodrugs and therapy were indicated. It made no sense then, and it still doesn't. While medications are taking effect, a psychiatrist can work psychotherapeutically with a patient he or she has already gotten to know. This seems more reasonable than the current managed-care strategy of splitting treatment between a therapist and a psychiatrist, particularly when there is good evidence that an integrated approach is more cost effective (Dewan 1999). Resist third-party payers trying to segment your mental health service into unnecessary slices. If you need psychodrugs *and* psychotherapy and you have found the right psychiatrist, insist on a single provider.

In summary, you want a psychiatrist who has mastered a variety of mind concepts, tools, and techniques and who is competent using them. Specific therapeutic approaches are not nearly as critical as a therapist's confidence in what he or she does (Frank and Frank 1991). Your psychiatrist should be able to use mind work aides ably and selectively—not according to a predetermined cookie-cutter approach, but as indicated by your special needs.

In the next chapter, I continue this discussion of mind work by reviewing other insightful sources.

CHAPTER SEVEN

Mind Work II

Windows into the Mind

- Choose a psychiatrist flexible of thought and personally responsive.

- Find one who is a good and fair negotiator.

- One who respects adaptive eccentricities.

- Supplement your psychiatric encounters with the experiences of others.

- Choose a psychiatrist who understands problems beyond diagnosis.

Working with mind problems demands a psychiatrist be able to treat, encourage, educate, motivate, confront, and support— and know when each is required. None of this is specific to any given diagnosis. Problems of mind cut across psychiatric diagnoses. All this is to say, look for a psychiatrist who keeps on learning and remains open to new approaches. For the complete psychiatrist, understanding how human behavior goes wrong and can be corrected becomes a lifelong study. Avoid the psychiatrist who has a pat answer for everything. Find one who values your particular story more than your diagnosis—one who is more consultative and less dogmatic as he or she focuses on your particular problems. And don't forget that although a complete psychiatrist has much to offer and can be extraordinarily helpful, it's still *your* life, *your* answers, and *your* solutions that ultimately matter. In the end, it's what you can embrace and live by that counts.

WINDOWS INTO THE MIND

Supplement your work with a psychiatrist by learning from the experiences of others such as found in personal memoirs, with their richness of material and the poignancy of first-person reporting. (Although books provide most of the supporting material in this chapter, increasingly, the Internet offers valuable resources. A list of particularly relevant websites appears in an appendix at the end of this book.)

In Kay Redfield Jamison's *An Unquiet Mind*, we meet a woman who eventually becomes a professor of psychiatry at Johns Hopkins and coauthor of an authoritative textbook on bipolar disorder—this after living much of her adult life as a "closeted bipolar." Her story has it all: denial, resistance to treatment, manic violence, suicidal depression, suicide attempts, lost loves, and other self-destructive behavior. Jamison's marvelous skills of self-observation and writing provide an added bonus. Listen to how she describes the double-edged sword of mania from inside: "When you're high it's tremendous. The ideas and feelings are fast and frequent like shooting stars. . . . Shyness goes, the right words, and gestures are suddenly there, the power to captivate others a felt certainty. . . . Sensuality is pervasive and the desire to seduce and be seduced irresistible. . . . But, somewhere, this changes. The fast ideas are far too fast, and there are far too many; overwhelming confusion replaces clarity" (Jamison 1995). Although Jamison eventually confronts her problem for what it is and accepts her need for lithium to prevent self-harm and life-disrupting mood swings, she provides a valuable insight into why manic persons often resist treatment. "Even when I have been most psychotic—delusional, hallucinating, frenzied—I have been aware of finding new corners in my mind and heart," she acknowledges. "Some of those corners were incredible and beautiful and took my breath away and made me feel as though I could die right then and the images would sustain me."

For a look at the suffocating, life-denying experience of deep depression, read *Darkness Visible: A Memoir of Madness*, written by William Styron. The Pulitzer Prize–winning novelist—author of *Sophie's Choice*, *The Confessions of Nat Turner*, and *Lie Down in Darkness*—recounts the "unfocused dread" he felt as he fell into a black hole of agitated depression and anxiety, contrasting it with the pain of a broken arm: "despair, owing to some evil trick played upon the sick brain by the inhabiting psyche, comes to resemble the diabolical discomfort of being imprisoned in a fiercely over-heated room. And because no breeze stirs this cauldron, because there is no escape from this smothering confinement, it is entirely natural that the victim begins to think ceaselessly of oblivion" (Styron 1990). Styron relates his hellish struggle with insomnia even as he becomes addicted to the sleep aid Halcion. He pulls no punches as he portrays his largely unsuccessful trials of psychotherapy, psychopharmacology, and psychiatric hospitalization and assesses his psychiatrist harshly.

"Nor could he say much of value to me. His platitudes were not Christian but, almost as ineffective, dicta drawn straight from the pages of *The Diagnostic and Statistical Manual of the American Psychiatric Association* . . . and the solace he offered me was an antidepressant medication called Ludiomil. The pill made me edgy, disagreeably hyperactive, and when the dosage was increased after ten days it blocked my bladder for hours one night." Looking back on his experience, Styron concludes: "seclusion and time" did the most good along with the "untiring and priceless" support of a friend (Styron 1990).

In his international best seller titled *The Noonday Demon*, Andrew Solomon provides a scholarly review along with his moving personal account of depression. He poignantly describes the terror of depression that leaves him longing for suicidal relief but too exhausted and drained to do it. "I knew then that I could never kill this vine of depression. . . . all I wanted was for it to let me die. But it had taken from me the energy I would have needed to kill myself, and it would not kill me. If my trunk was rotting, this thing that fed on it was now too strong to let it fall. . . . Every second of being alive hurt me. Because this thing had drained all fluid from me, I could not even cry" (Solomon 2001).

Novels, movies, and short stories also serve as valuable psychiatric sources. I've never forgotten a medical school experience when a gifted psychoanalyst used Ernest Hemmingway's "Short Happy Life of Francis McCumber" to illustrate a tragic power struggle between a husband and wife that eventually ends in "unintentional" homicide. Later I found valuable psychiatric insights in other short stories. Dorothy Parker's "Big Blonde" portrays a woman on a neurotic merry-go-round, stuck in a recurring pattern of self-destructive behavior, and Lawrence

Sargent Hall's "The Ledge" tells a sparse but heart-wrenching, existential story of heroism and youthful vulnerability played out in the face of oblivion.

For years William Tucker, a psychiatrist affiliated with John Hopkins, has presented short stories to colleagues as "case histories." In his collection *How People Change*, he explains his approach this way: "Why is empathy not enough in itself to understand our patients? In theory it should be, but in reality most of us physicians simply have not had many of these life experiences . . . there are limits to our comprehension, limits that the great writers have transcended" (Tucker 2007).

I also consider of great value the writings of sensitive journalists who explore mental disability and treatment. Former *Newsweek* journalist Peter Wyden, in his book *Conquering Schizophrenia: A Father, His Son, and a Medical Breakthrough*, recounts twenty-five years of his son's tortuous, heartbreaking experiences with mental health treatment after suffering a psychotic break in his twenties. In all, the son saw more than fifty different doctors, some terrific, others not so good. Based on interviews with patients, administrators, psychiatrists, and researchers, Wyden details a bittersweet tale of a chaotic mental health care world, plagued by conflicting opinions regarding psychiatric treatment and diagnosis, bureaucratic bungling, and contorted mental health laws. At the book's conclusion, his son seems improved on a new drug, olanzepine (Zyprexa), a drug that subsequently would be found to cause serious weight gain and diabetes (Wyden 1998).

If you choose to go deeper into the nature of mind work, check out Irvin Yalom's *The Gift of Therapy* (Yalom 2002). This gem of a book is filled with nuggets of wisdom from a psychiatrist who has spent much of his professional life practicing and studying psychotherapy. It is not a theory book but more a discussion of nuts-and-bolts matters of psychotherapy as suggested by the various chapter titles: "Engage the Patient," "Let the Patient Matter to You," "Create a New Therapy for Each Patient," "Acknowledge Your Errors," "Provide Feedback Effectively," "Never (Almost Never) Make Decisions for Patients," "Talk About Life Meaning," etcetera. This book would be valuable preparation for anyone going into therapy, and it provides a good look at many of the things you should expect from a complete psychiatrist.

Much of what I've learned about clinical psychiatry, however, has not come from reading books or listening to lectures, but rather from patients themselves. I'll never forget an older woman, elegant in appearance, who came to me years ago following months of grieving the death of her companion of many years. At the conclusion of our third or fourth session she graciously thanked me and explained that we were finished. What I could do for her, I had done, she said with a grateful smile. "There are so many things you don't know—you can't know—at your age," she whispered, "and I don't have the time or energy to tell you." She warmly shook my hand before leaving. "Thank you for your help," she said. There are things your psychiatrist will not understand, regardless of how good he or she is. Humility is always in order. It's an important trait to look for in a psychiatrist.

VALUING ECCENTRICITY

Patients have taught me respect for eccentric lives.

I am often reminded of this truth when I play my favorite golf course. On numerous occasions I have watched a gray-haired gentleman, slowed by years and well defended from the hot Texas sun by a broad-brimmed hat and a long-sleeve white shirt, slowly take his position teeing off. If you weren't familiar with this man, his rickety appearance would make you groan inside as you await disaster. And as though to confirm your worst fears, this ancient golfer tortuously winds up Rube Goldberg fashion, defiant of all hallowed golfing principles, before delivering the clubhead square to the ball and watching it fly down the middle of the fairway 180 yards. *Eccentricity is not an automatic disqualifier from living a meaningful life.* Many successful adaptations—quirky, if not outright bizarre—fall outside the boundaries of "normal." They relate to where people live, how they spend their time, how they comport themselves, what they believe, what they think and feel, and how they relate to other people. Some psychiatrists make the mistake of equating eccentricity with illness. You want a psychiatrist who recognizes successful adaptation when he sees it. Locking onto symptoms as nothing more than *DSM* criteria belies respect for unusual lives that don't fit the norms but are adaptive.

The author and neurologist Oliver Sacks describes persons with severe neurological problems struggling against all odds. In one of his books Sacks recounts the plight of a crime novelist who, because of a brain injury, becomes unable to read despite his continuing ability to write (Sacks 2010). Unwilling to accept this loss, the man comes up with an ingenious way to read by tracing words with his tongue on the back of his teeth. In effect he was reading again by writing. Persons with severe mental disabilities make similar adaptations that too often go unrecognized for what they are. With the right kind of help, many are able to capitalize on other strengths enough to compensate for what otherwise would be overwhelming deficits. It would be helpful if psychiatrists—and other mental health professionals as well—emphasized patient strengths more and deficits and diagnosis less; if they were more supportive of nonconforming behaviors as acceptable alternatives; and if they construed symptoms as important but not the whole story. Look for one like this.

As I come to the end of these comments on mind work, I want to emphasize one point. Mind work has its limits; not all mind problems are best explained psychologically. They sometimes arise from harsh demands in life. Particularly for persons with severe mental and emotional problems, some of life's greatest challenges concern basic necessities. Many of these individuals live socially isolated, poverty-stricken lives. Housing is often marginal, transportation an ongoing problem. Obtaining appropriate medical care becomes difficult. These persons are often high risk for assault and addiction. They live on the edge of catastrophe struggling to navigate bureaucratic labyrinths such as Social Security, Medicaid, and federal Section 8 housing. They sometimes struggle with ruthless board and care operators, negligent landlords, and even conservators who rip them off. They go through tedious, red-tape-ridden processes obtaining SSI *before* they can receive job training and other supportive services. And once a person receives SSI, powerful incentives kick in to encourage their remaining dependent and not working, even if they are able (Turkewitz and Linderman 2012).

Over the past half century, psychiatric patients have left state hospitals with the promise of better community care only to find resources sucked away and hospital doors closed. Thousands find themselves on the streets, homeless and with inadequate services. Increasingly, many end up in jails and prisons, where they receive pitiful, if any, treatment.

Persons with persisting mental disorders also risk extreme social isolation. Interpersonal relationships, while difficult at times, provide much of what is most meaningful in life. Less well recognized is the powerful influence they exert on both physical and mental health. Several decades ago I worked with a talented group of people designing a California statewide public health campaign named Friends Can Be Good Medicine. The intent was to raise public awareness about the health consequences of inadequate social support: shortened lives and a host of medical and psychological problems (House et al. 1988). As a health risk, lack of social support ranks with high cholesterol, obesity, and hypertension. The chaotic social lives of patients with severe mental disability often go inadequately addressed by psychiatrists and mental health care programs. Such problems require more than psychotherapy. And more than psychodrugs.

Extradiagnostic considerations such as these are creatively addressed by what has been called the "recovery model." One of its most articulate spokespersons, Mark Ragins, a psychiatrist and founding member of the Village (Integrated Service Agency) in Long Beach, California, describes four critical aspects of mental health recovery: regaining hope, acquiring a renewed sense of self-efficacy, accepting self-responsibility, and reestablishing a meaningful life. The recovery approach is person (not diagnosis) focused and considers meaningful lives the primary objective. While supportive of traditional treatments, the recovery approach emphasizes help with a host of real-life problems that go beyond diagnosis.

Successful recovery programs like the Village recognize the great value of employment in keeping psychiatric patients out of the hospital. When I was a resident in psychiatry, Dr. David Daniels, a Stanford University psychiatrist, created

Dan Services, a pioneering job-provider company for veterans with mental disabilities. Much of the work made available to patients came from contracts Daniels and his team secured for assembling electronic components. Patients employed in those jobs fared much better than those who remained unemployed. Other work initiatives have shown similar results—programs such as Fountain House, Inc., in New York and Fairweather Lodges scattered across the country. Employment is not possible for all patients with severe disabilities but when it is, this aspect of recovery makes a crucial difference. What I have never understood is why supportive employment programs like these are not a standard service in all mental health programs. As it is, most of them neglect employment as a recovery tool.

In summary, you need a psychiatrist who is expert at prescribing psychodrugs when they are required, but also one competent at mind work. A psychiatrist who can help you better understand yourself, the role you play in your troubled story, and the misguided patterns and irrational fears that upset your life; one who listens well and focuses more on you than on your diagnosis; one who respects *adaptive* eccentricities and is willing to explore the meaning of symptoms as well as controlling them when they are dysfunctional; and one who recognizes mind problems that are more sociocultural than psychological in nature. In addition you can supplement your work with a psychiatrist by pursuing information from other sources that provide you with compelling windows into the world and problems of mind.

CHAPTER EIGHT

Finding the Right Psychiatrist

As I'm sure you can see, psychiatry's predicament complicates finding the right psychiatrist. Despite academic talk about a bright new day, clinical psychiatry trudges along, mindless with a fading medical identity, holding tight to questionable diagnoses, obsessed with phantom chemical imbalances, and equipped with a tired collection of modestly effective psychodrugs. With universal health insurance on its way and with the pressing need to train more primary care physicians, we may not be too far away from a serious rethinking of the use of limited medical school slots to train psychiatrists.

PSYCHIATRY'S FUTURE

I wonder how the Las Vegas bookies would size up psychiatry's future. What would they predict if asked the odds of one of the following four scenarios over the next twenty years: (1) After a series of major brain science breakthroughs, psychiatry goes to the head of the class, a bona fide medical specialty, increasingly able to match psychiatric conditions with brain/ body alterations and to treat them with advanced psychodrugs, brain stimulation, immunizations, and genetic engineering. (2) Without any major scientific breakthroughs, psychiatry— still depending on a stable of me-too psychodrugs—barely hangs on, a medical specialty in name only, performing mainly routine "med checks." (3) Hit by the push for greater health-care efficiency, psychiatry becomes a defunct specialty after being squeezed out by lesser-trained professionals. (4) Psychiatry resurrects itself by renewing its medical skills, scaling back its overdependence on psychodrugs, and embracing problems of the mind and mind/body, thereby enabling the discipline to emerge as a distinctive psychosomatic medical specialty.

If you listen to leaders of psychiatry, you might think number 1 is in the bag. And, of course, they could be right. But, personally, I think it highly unlikely that brain science breakthroughs will help psychiatrists anytime soon. If neuroscience discoveries were going to transform psychiatry, we would already see the evidence. On the other hand, given managed care's grip on health-care policy, number 3 seems a distinct possibility. From a strictly cost perspective, psychiatry holds a poor hand. In a cheapest-is-best health-care climate, being the highest-priced mental health professional cannot be a good thing.

By now you know my preference for psychiatry's future. I'm pulling for number 4 (a re-emergence of psychiatry with equal emphasis on mind, body, and brain). I think it the most viable, relevant, and professionally rewarding scenario. But if you push me, if you insist I go with my head rather than my heart, I bet number 2 the most likely outcome. Institutional inertia being what it is, psychiatry probably muddles along, relegated mainly to performing med checks and writing up mindless evaluations that meet all the regulatory requirements. My reason for betting this way, sad to say, relates mainly to the power of psychodrug makers to maintain the status quo. The drug makers have the money; their influence remains pervasive. For decades, these companies have been hugely successful selling mediocre psychodrugs in the absence of any major advances. That's impressive! And with their extensive penetration into research, academic, and clinical psychiatry as well as into the discipline's major publications and national organization (APA), I don't see them losing their domination anytime soon. If they do, it will only be because young psychiatrists and their patients finally get fed up with chemical imbalance psychiatry. Psychiatry has a lot of work to do to reclaim its position as a deserving medical discipline.

AVOIDING THE WRONG PSYCHIATRIST

But regardless of the discipline's bleak future, if you look carefully, there will always be the right psychiatrist for you. Your challenge is to avoid the wrong ones. Make sure you don't end up with a burned-out, disgruntled psychiatrist, one with no passion for what he or she does. Typically, this is the psychiatrist with no sense of humor, the one who goes through the motions, watches the clock, has little to say, and appears to have trouble keeping track of where you left off from session to session.

Avoid psychiatrists who don't listen. You want a psychiatrist who carefully follows what you are saying and takes time to clarify what he or she doesn't understand, one who routinely asks if you have questions and, when you do, answers them to your satisfaction.

Steer clear of the psychiatrist who overemphasizes your diagnosis. It's much more important that he or she understand you—your particular problems, history, and symptoms—and fashion your treatment accordingly. Similarly, reject the psychiatrist who explains every problem as needing psychodrugs.

Avoiding psychiatrists with these traits does not guarantee you will find the right psychiatrist, but it gives you a fighting chance. Keep this in mind: comparisons between psychotherapy and psychodrug treatment, particularly for nonpsychotic symptoms, repeatedly show the two modalities in a dead heat. As for which of the two provides the longer-lasting benefit, evidence gives a slight advantage to psychotherapy. One analysis showed that depressed patients treated with psychotherapy had less depression than patients taking antidepressant medication, and the longer the follow-up, the greater the difference (deMaat et al. 2006).

KNOWING WHAT YOU ARE LOOKING FOR

Respect the central importance of your psychiatrist's personality. Personality might not be a huge consideration if you were looking for a brain surgeon, but it's of utmost relevance when you choose a psychiatrist. You want someone personable and flexible who exhibits common sense; someone with a sense of humor who can make you smile and lighten up even in the darkest of times. One who understands that in the overall scheme of things seldom are problems as serious as they seem. You want a psychiatrist who is a good teacher and takes the necessary time to educate you about your problems and your treatment.

Choose a respectful psychiatrist. One who doesn't keep you waiting for long periods and doesn't cancel appointments at the last moment. One who's willing for you to disagree and choose courses of action he or she may question.

For sure you want a psychiatrist who is expert at prescribing psychodrugs. One who prescribes them judiciously and uses the least number of psychodrugs at the lowest dosages necessary. A psychiatrist committed to the crucial importance of tapering medications slowly and, when you no longer need them, stopping them altogether. One who is aware of the potential risks of long-term uninterrupted use.

Choose a psychiatrist who—while he or she considers diagnosis—thinks beyond it, using it only as a guide, aware it may mislead more than help. Choose one who sees you as a person with a unique story that defies standard treatment protocols; one who is not satisfied simply "treating" your problems but, instead, insists on educating you so that you become more adept at anticipating problems and handling them yourself. In short, you want an artisan psychiatrist who uses various tools and skills to help you become your own therapist.

Be sure your psychiatrist remains a competent physician. You should be able to trust that he or she will correctly identify medical problems that aggravate your psychiatric problems and recognize medial conditions that masquerade, including adverse medication effects.

In addition to being a physician and expert on psychodrugs, the complete psychiatrist appreciates the world of mind and the importance of story. He or she talks to you in language you understand and encourages you to imagine solutions you have not thought of. This psychiatrist helps you see the role you play in your own problems and understand better ways of dealing with your situation as opposed to singularly focusing on extinguishing your symptoms. He or she respects the social and economic barriers that persons with severe mental and emotional problems confront on a daily basis and advocates for relief whenever possible.

The best psychiatrists are those who learn from the past, even from possible mistakes. From my own career, three patients quickly come to mind.

An older man I saw in a walk-in crisis service. Grieving over his dead wife, he said. Couldn't sleep, mind racing. No previous psychiatric care. There was little more to go on, and there were patients to see on the inpatient service upstairs. A hastily written two-week script for Seroquel and a return appointment had to suffice. And then a few days later, an official notification of death. The man had returned home and, with a liquor bottle in one hand and the pills I had prescribed in the other, proceeded to kill himself with a drawn-out overdose and a hard-liquor chaser. If I had taken more time would I have sensed what was about to happen? Would I have picked up on the hopelessness and guilt this man likely felt. No way of really knowing now, but still sometimes his image comes to me. I think about how I might have handled things differently.

A middle-aged woman with two children, angry at her husband's leaving her for a younger woman. She said she was depressed but "not suicidal." Eventually, when I confronted her about her excessive drinking, she dropped out of treatment. Several months later, an item in the local paper described her careful preparation attempting to seal off the air vents to the rest of her house. Later, as the car ran in the garage, a hose carried the exhaust through the car window while her two young children slept in their upstairs bedroom. Tragically, despite her best efforts, they were found dead in their beds, also victims of the exhaust gas that had crept up the inside wall of the garage and spilled over into the ventilation system. Would it have turned out differently if I had not confronted her so hard about her drinking? Was the timing wrong? Did it keep me from giving her the support she needed to deal with her life falling apart? The memory of this woman raises a lot of questions for me.

And, finally, a young man brought in as a case of intoxicated schizophrenia—a mistaken diagnosis, as it turned out. He had no history of schizophrenic symptoms. What he did have were complex seizures since childhood. Recently, when he had run out of medication and was unable to pay for more, his seizures had returned. This was what had caused him to become confused, unsteady, and bizarre and led to his misdiagnosis. With this information in hand I stopped his antipsychotic and restarted his seizure medication. Within forty-eight hours the young man was a different person. His thoughts were clear, his mood upbeat. Understandably, he was anxious to leave the hospital and get on with his life. But the blood level of his seizure medication remained low. I called his general doctor, who was set to follow him for his seizure problem. We talked. The doctor said he preferred going slow with anticonvulsant dosing. I should send the young man home, and he would see him the following week. It seemed a reasonable plan. The patient's parents, out from the East Coast, were thrilled to see their son fully recovered. They also pressed for his release. Done. But a few days later, word came, he had been found dead—sitting at his kitchen table, pills scattered on the floor. My first thought was suicide. But he hadn't been depressed, and the coroner found no sign of an overdose; instead, he concluded the patient had died from an uninterrupted series of seizures. What would have happened had I kept him in the hospital for a few more days, enough time for his seizure medication to become fully effective? Would it have made the difference?

The good psychiatrist resists putting tragic cases like these out of mind; rather, he or she embraces them, making certain to learn as much as possible for future patients. It's the least we can do.

OPEN TO THE FUTURE

Finally, let me encourage you to find a psychiatrist open to new, nonmedication technologies. Years ago I wrote a paper with a colleague titled "The Self-Education of Psychiatric Residents" (Taylor and Torrey 1972). It championed self-directed education: individualized training based on the specific interests, abilities, and needs of individual residents. From this perspective, the academic psychiatrist—as opposed to being the repository of all psychiatric knowledge—served more as a facilitator, directing residents in their own self-education programs, connecting them with resources, and providing them with appropriate training experiences. Years later, I still think self-education essential for psychiatrists, perhaps even more so. My advice to you is to find a psychiatrist obsessed with continuing to learn.

The explosion in communication technologies creates intriguing possibilities for psychiatry. Computer-assisted psychotherapy has become a reality. Cell phone apps are now used as treatment aids. E-mail serves as a physician extender. Cognitive-behavioral therapy is delivered online for depression and anxiety (Spek et al. 2007). Virtual reality deconditioning helps patients with severe phobias and post-traumatic stress (Rothbaum et al. 2000; Difede et al. 2007).

Thanks to the amazing speed and power of modern computers, persons can now interact with virtual humans (or non-humans) and inhabit avatars of themselves (Lanier 2010).

Imagine a schoolkid being taught about animal life—say, that of a lobster—by temporarily turning into one! In an article titled, "In Cybertherapy, Avatars Assist with Healing," *New York Times* journalist Benedict Carey reports some of these emerging treatment possibilities: "Researchers are populating digital worlds with autonomous, virtual humans that can evoke the same tensions as in real-life encounters. People with social anxiety are struck dumb when asked questions by a virtual stranger. Heavy drinkers feel strong urges to order something from a virtual bartender, while gamblers are drawn to sit down and join a group playing on virtual slot machines. And therapists can engage patients at the very moment those sensations are felt" (Carey 2010a). A recent treatment program in London taught sixteen persons with schizophrenia how to construct a computer-animated avatar with faces they chose and digital voices that resembled the "voices" they were troubled by. They were encouraged to interact with the avatar—even challenge it. Their therapists responded using the avatar's voice, which gradually changed from persecuting to supportive. After six weeks all the patients reported that their hallucinated "voices" had become less intense and less disturbing. Three of them stopped having hallucinations altogether and three months later were still symptom free. One of these patients had been hearing "voices" persistently for sixteen years (Luhrmann 2013).

Virtual therapists are now being used. A pilot study at the University of Quebec tracked two groups of patients who suffered from social anxiety. One group saw a psychotherapist weekly for fourteen weeks; the other group interacted with a "virtual" therapist over the same period. Both groups improved much more than persons kept on a treatment waiting list (Carey 2010a). In an earlier article, Carey described a three-foot-tall robot (developed by the University of Southern California) used to treat a six-year-old autistic boy. As a companion, the robot maintained eye contact, imitated the boy, and took turns (Carey 2010b). Robotic animals have proven to exert a calming influence on persons with dementia. Internet social-networking sites are exploding, and in some version may prove useful helping with the social isolation experienced by many mentally disabled patients.

Find a psychiatrist who follows the emergence of new treatments. Take, for example, the use of an antibiotic to treat psychotic conditions. Minocycline is a tetracycline antibiotic with powerful anti-inflammatory action, presumably the basis for the neuroprotection the drug provides persons with Parkinson's and Huntington's diseases (Thomas, Dong, et al. 2003). Minocycline has also proven beneficial as treatment for acute schizophrenic psychosis. After taking this antibiotic for infections, two patients experienced dramatic improvement in their psychotic symptoms only to deteriorate once the medication was stopped. When it was restarted, the psychoses resolved again (Miyaoka et al. 2007). This outcome has been followed up with a larger number of patients. "Robust" clinical improvement was reported for both positive and negative symptoms (Miyaoka et al. 2008). The psychiatrist you want is one who follows such developments with interest and makes considered judgments about when to use them and when to wait; one who understands how to weigh early promising results against the severity and persistence of symptoms and the possibility of adverse effects. You want a psychiatrist willing to suggest a nutrition supplement instead of a psychodrug when there's good evidence it will give you similar benefit.

Undoubtedly, future psychiatric treatment will include emerging somatic therapies. Growing evidence supports a role for acupuncture in its various forms—manual, electrical, and laser based—in depression. Adverse effects are minimal (Wu et al. 2012). Transcranial magnetic stimulation (TMS) represents another promising antidepressant therapy. This procedure involves the application of a device to the scalp through which pulsed magnetic waves are directed at the frontal areas of the brain. Sessions lasting approximately forty minutes are administered daily for four to six weeks. Thus far, results are modest. A few patients do extremely well while others experience little if any benefit, but there appear to be no serious adverse effects (George et al. 2010).

My advice is this: consider such a somatic treatment *only* after discussing it with your psychiatrist so that you fully understand the rationale, the effectiveness, and the side effects, both short and long term. Unfortunately, the history of psychiatric somatic therapies is clouded. Treatments such as insulin coma, progressive electroconvulsive therapy, and prefrontal lobotomy—all were initially touted as extremely effective and without complications. Sadly, experience proved otherwise. Caution is advised.

I hope I've convinced you to be *assertive* finding a psychiatrist. This is not a decision you should make simply on the recommendation of friends or even a doctor. By its nature, selecting a psychiatrist is more complicated than choosing a general doctor. To be sure, technical competency remains a central issue, but there's also the psychiatrist's personality and the personal chemistry between the two of you. If you take time to think through the kind of psychiatrist you want, you are better prepared to make the choice. Still, there will always be a subjective element. Even if a psychiatrist comes with highest commendation and impressive diplomas and certificates, respect your instincts. If after a few sessions, the relationship doesn't feel right, move on.

This is not to say there won't be times when your psychiatrist points out things you would rather not hear. In those moments treatment may be difficult, but you'll get through it if you are comfortable with your psychiatrist and trust him or her enough to keep working. This is what makes the therapeutic psychiatric relationship so vital.

As a discerning consumer—knowledgeable about what's covered in this book—you are better prepared to find the right psychiatrist. If you suffer from chronic symptoms that require ongoing psychiatric contact, demand that the sessions be more than token med checks. If your treatment involves psychodrugs, require a full explanation of why you need them. Insist on the fewest medications necessary and the lowest effective doses. Regardless of your diagnosis, do not automatically accept that you need psychodrugs for the rest of your life. Periodically, raise the possibility of tapering off medications on a trial basis.

Resist continuing to see your psychiatrist simply because it becomes routine. It's perfectly acceptable that you ask for more or less contact as your situation changes. And, when your work is finished, bid your psychiatrist good-bye. Even patients who experience ongoing psychiatric problems should consider temporary breaks from their psychiatrist. He or she will be there when you return ready to resume your care. If you are a person seeking psychiatric help for a crisis in your life, embrace the idea that your work will be time limited. When you have clarified your problems, changed what you can, accepted what you have no control over, experienced a lessening of symptoms, and sense your work is finished, avoid hanging on. Inquire about stopping treatment. If your psychiatrist disagrees, insist he or she explain why. What remains to be done, how it will be accomplished, and approximately how much more time it will take? When you are convinced you no longer need psychiatric care—even if it's only a break—let yourself feel the satisfaction of a finished task. The complete psychiatrist will celebrate with you, wish you well, and assure you that, if ever again you should need his service, he will welcome you back, knowing you more as a unique person than a psychiatric diagnosis.

SUMMARY QUESTIONS
& ANSWERS

QUESTION 1: Finding the right psychiatrist becomes an issue only if you need one. *What are major reasons for seeing a psychiatrist?*

ANSWERS:

- A first-time severe disturbance in mood, thought, or behavior, especially if this change occurs "out of the blue" with no obvious stressor.
- Intense psychological symptoms—depression or anxiety, suicidal thoughts, panic attacks, bizarre behavior, psychotic experiences such as hallucinations or delusional thought—that become life disrupting.
- An acute onset of mental or behavioral problems paired with unexplained physical symptoms such as impaired speech or impaired balance.
- When psychodrug treatment becomes a consideration after therapy or counseling fails to provide relief.
- The re-emergence of a psychiatric problem that has required psychodrug treatment in the past.
- Psychiatric symptoms complicated by serious medical problems.
- Need for counseling or therapy when you know of a psychiatrist said to be, by people you trust, outstanding and likely superior to other options.
- An ongoing, severe psychiatric condition clearly unresponsive to treatments other than psychodrugs.

QUESTION 2: Persons who go to mental health professionals often do so with few expectations. *What reasonable expectations should you have of your psychiatrist?*

ANSWERS:

- More interested in your unique story and problems than an official psychiatric diagnosis.
- Open to working on mind problems as well as prescribing psychodrugs when indicated.
- Willing to take the time needed to explain your problems and treatment options in terms you understand.
- A competent physician.

QUESTION 3: A psychiatrist's personality plays a critical role in psychiatric treatment. *What are some of the most important personal characteristics of the right psychiatrist?*

ANSWERS:

- Professional in conduct.
- Personable, empathetic, flexible, and respectful.
- A good listener.
- Has confidence that inspires your trust, but is open to your ideas and objections.
- Creative in his or her ability to fashion treatment specific for you.

QUESTION 4: Although overemphasized, psychodrugs are sometimes essential treatment tools. *What are good reasons for considering psychiatric medications?*

ANSWERS:

- Lack of success with therapy or counseling.
- Severe disabling symptoms that threaten to disrupt your life.
- A history of similar symptoms that have required psychodrugs for resolution.

- A history of psychosis that relentlessly recurs in the absence of psychodrugs.

QUESTION 5: If you take psychodrugs, *what are some guiding principles for their use?*

ANSWERS:

- Use when alternatives are not available or not effective.
- Only as long as they are needed.
- The fewest number possible.
- At the lowest effective dose.
- With periodic attempts to stop (always *slowly* tapered).
- Use for extended, uninterrupted periods only when you and your psychiatrist are fully convinced you cannot function without them.

QUESTION 6: The official list of psychiatric diagnoses grows relentlessly longer. Diagnoses are required for billing and regulatory purposes, but for patients, too often, they remain mystifying labels that mislead more than they enlighten. *What are the characteristics and implications of psychiatric diagnoses?*

ANSWERS:

- Despite their appearance of being precise, objective categories, psychiatric diagnoses most often are applied to broad spectrums of troublesome changes in mood, thinking, and behavior.
- Unlike medical diagnoses, they are not supported by biomarkers such as lab tests.
- Symptoms associated with various diagnoses often overlap.
- Officially, diagnoses remain the target of treatment despite there being no known causes of psychiatric disorders.
- Clinically, they are less important than your particular problems, situation, history, and symptoms.

- They mislead when they are construed as implying that persons with similar diagnoses are more alike than different.
- Psychiatric diagnoses encourage mental health care providers, including psychiatrists, to view and treat patients more as "cases" than as individuals with unique problems who happen to share common symptoms.

QUESTION 7: Increasingly, psychiatrists are losing their skills and knowledge of general medicine. *What are the most important reasons you should choose a psychiatrist who remains a competent physician?*

ANSWERS:

- Recognition of medical conditions that masquerade as psychiatric symptoms.
- Understanding of how medical conditions aggravate psychiatric symptoms and vice versa.
- Sensitivity to adverse side effects of psychodrugs and other medications.
- Facility for bridging mind and body in psychiatric assessment and treatment.
- Familiarity with medical complications of substance addictions and with medications useful as aids in addiction treatment.

QUESTION 8: Compared with the rest of medicine, psychiatry serves as a unique political lighting rod, particularly as it interfaces with the law and social policy. *How might the politics of psychiatry affect you?*

ANSWERS:

- Risk of stigma sometimes associated with mental and emotional conditions.

- Narrowing of treatment options due to the overshadowing influence of psychodrug makers on psychiatric treatment.
- Risk of inadequate legal representation when dealing with mental health law.
- Loss of certain civil liberties if held involuntarily for psychiatric problems.

QUESTION 9: Psychiatric conditions are often said to be caused by *chemical imbalances* in the brain. *What does this mean in terms of your treatment?*

ANSWERS:

- "Chemical imbalance" is a marketing term, not a scientific explanation.
- No specific chemical imbalances are associated with psychiatric disorders.
- Chemical changes (neurotransmitters) produced by psychodrugs provide symptom relief *without* correcting a fanciful underlying imbalance.
- As a term, "chemical imbalance" misleads by pushing aside other significant contributing factors in a person's life.

QUESTION 10: Mind problems arising from difficulties in living often lead to troublesome changes in mood, behavior, or thought. *What is mind work?*

ANSWERS:

- Therapeutic explorations of your life story:
- Specifically focused on your particular situation, symptoms, and history.
- Creatively forged out of the therapeutic relationship and various concepts, tools, and strategies appropriate for you.

- Aimed at helping you successfully integrate what you are going through into your ongoing life story in preparation for the future.
- Compatible with the simultaneous use of psychodrugs when appropriate.

QUESTION 11: Finding a psychiatrist is not something you want to do through the Yellow Pages. *How would you go about identifying the right psychiatrist for you?*

ANSWERS:

- Use the website of your state medical board to establish that a psychiatrist has a medical license and is in good standing.
- Check with your insurance or managed care provider to see if there are restrictions as to which psychiatrist you choose.
- Ask people you respect if they know of psychiatrists they would recommend. You might ask, for example, your doctor, minister, or lawyer, even a mental health professional—perhaps someone you have seen before—or a good friend.
- Recall if you have ever read about or heard a presentation by a psychiatrist who impressed you.
- Understand that while this kind of background work will be helpful, it will not be enough to make your final choice.
- Be prepared by knowing what you are looking for.
- Accept that the first psychiatrist you consult may not be the one for you.

QUESTION 12: Unfortunately, finding the right psychiatrist becomes more complicated because of special rules and restrictions imposed by your insurance or managed care company. *What are common obstacles you might encounter?*

Answers:

- As a way of being more profitable some insurance/managed care companies restrict your selection to a panel of preapproved psychiatrists.
- Some will insist you see a lesser-trained professional first.
- Some will arbitrarily restrict how many times you see a psychiatrist.
- Some will insist you split your time, seeing a psychiatrist for psychodrugs and a therapist or counselor for therapy.
- Best strategy: Clarify in your mind why you need a psychiatrist and press your case. (It never hurts to have your general doctor support your need for a psychiatrist.)

APPENDIX

Medical News Today

www.medicalnewstoday.com

Provides hourly health news—including mental health matters—from respected sources such as the *Lancet, Journal of the American Medical Association (JAMA)*, and the *British Medical Journal* as well as articles written by the *Medical News Today* news team. Excellent search engine. Allows you to peruse whatever mental health subjects you choose. Results appear in chronological order, most recent items first. Standing "news categories" include *mental health* with specific listings for schizophrenia, bipolar disorder, ADHD, alcohol/addiction/drugs, psychology/psychiatry, food intolerance, and complementary (alternative) medicine. You can also search for nondiagnostic, nonmedication topics. For example, when I typed in "dreams," twenty items appeared. For "stress" there were two hundred listings.

National Institute of Mental Health

www.nimh.nih.gov

Good source of information on mental health research and mental disorders. Various diagnoses are listed with easy-to-navigate "quick links" to descriptions, signs and symptoms, treatment, and clinical trials. There is also news of clinical studies as well as articles by leading mental health professionals and scientists.

You can access various publications (many in Spanish) that can be read online, downloaded, or obtained free as hard copy.

Healthline

www.healthline.com

General-purpose health site with excellent mental health information. On the home page, the question "How Can We Help You Today?" appears. You simply type in your topic. For example, if you enter "depression," you will be able to conduct a general search or a more specific one on related subjects: symptoms, treatment, drug search. There's even a pill identifier. In addition there's coverage of a variety of general health and wellness topics as "featured topic centers."

PubMed Central (National Center for Biotechnology Information)

www.ncbi-nlm.nih.gov/pmc

This site is sponsored by the U.S. National Library of Medicine. It gives you access to extensive findings from research supported by the National Institutes of Health. Particularly good for information on specific psychiatric medications and their side effects. Start with *PMC Overview*. You can then search any topic you wish by typing in the name. Be prepared for an extensive number of listings.

MHA Village, A Program of Mental Health America of Los Angeles

www.mhavillage.org

The Village opened in 1990 as a pilot program based on a recovery model that emphasizes elements of care beyond diagnosis and routine psychodrugs. The Village—its work and website—has special relevance for persons who suffer with persistent mental/ emotional problems. I have included this listing primarily for the access it provides to the collected writings (*Exploring Recovery*) of Mark Ragins, a psychiatrist who has played a key role in evolving this exceptional program. The following is a selected list: "Let's Include Psychiatrists" (1993), "Partners in Medication Collaboration" (1993), "Thoughtful Psychopharmacology" (2005), "An Overview of the Village" (2008), "14 Things You Can Do to Rebuild Your Life" (2010).

National Mental Health Association
www.nmha.org

Provides mental health information by audience (women, older adults, friends and loved ones, etc.), by issue (anxiety, depression, grief and bereavement, etc.), and by disorder (bipolar, borderline personality, schizophrenia, panic disorder, etc.). There is also access to experts and media highlights covering various mental health issues. You will find discussions of the different mental health providers including psychiatrists, psychologists, mental health and drug counselors, clinical social workers, and pastoral counselors. Overviews are included of various treatments including self-help and support groups, with information on how to connect with various resources.

NAMI (National Alliance on Mental Illness)
www.nami.org

Sponsored by the nation's largest mental advocacy group, this website has four main sections: mental illness, education, support, and advocacy. You can search various mental health topics and keep abreast of clinical treatment trials that are searching

for participants. Also, the site provides discussion groups on
mental health topics and—if you are interested—facilitates your
joining NAMI. (There are also state branch websites for NAMI.)

WebMD
www.webmd.com
This is a well-organized general health-care site with extensive
information across the health spectrum including mental health
topics. Included is a "symptom checker," a drugs and medication center, and a health A–Z section that allows you to find
your topic alphabetically. Once you select a topic, a "center"
appears that provides an overview, discussions of diagnosis and
treatment, and a guide for finding help. Latest headlines, top
stories, discussions, and expert blogs are also included.

REFERENCES

Amen, Daniel. 2010. *Change Your Brain, Change Your Body*. New York: Three Rivers Press.

American Psychiatric Association. 2000. *Diagnostic and Statistical Manual of Mental Disorders*. 4th ed. Text Revision (*DSM-IV-TR*). Washington, DC: American Psychiatric Press.

———. 2013. *Diagnostic and Statistical Manual of Mental Disorders*. 5th ed. Washington, DC: American Psychiatric Press.

Amminger, G., M. Schafer, and K. Papageorgiou. 2010. Long-chain W-3 fatty acids for indicated prevention of psychotic disorders. *Archives of General Psychiatry* 67: 146–154.

Andersohn, Frank, Rene Schade, Sammy Suissa, et al. 2009. Long-term use of antidepressants for depressive disorders and the risk of diabetes mellitus. *American Journal of Psychiatry*, April 1 (online).

Angell, Marcia. 2004. The truth about the drug companies. *New York Review of Books*, July 15.

———. 2011a. The epidemic of mental illness: Why? *New York Review of Books*, June 23.

———. 2011b. The illusions of psychiatry. *New York Review of Books*, July 14.

AOL News. 2010. Big changes proposed for Bible of psychiatric treatment. February 10.

Aronson, Eliot, and Judson Mills, 1959. The effect of severity of initiation on liking for a group. *Journal of Abnormal and Social Psychology* 59: 177–181.

Babyak, Michael, James Blumenthal, and Steve Herman. 2000. Exercise treatment for major depression: Maintenance of therapeutic benefit at 10 months. *Psychosomatic Medicine* 62: 633–638.

Barden, N., J. Reul, and F. Holsboer. 1995. Do antidepressants stabilize mood through actions on the hypothalamic-pituitary-adrenalcortical system? *Trends in Neurosciences* 18: 6–11.

Begley, Sharon. 2010. The depressing news about antidepressants. *Newsweek* (February 8): 34–37, 39–41.

———. 2013. Psychiatrists unveil their long-awaited diagnostic "bible." Reuters, May 17.

Behzadi, A., Z. Omrani, M. Chalian, et al. 2009. Folic acid efficacy as an alternative drug added to sodium valproate in the treatment of acute phase of mania in bipolar disorder: A double-blind randomized controlled trial. *ACTA Psychiatrica Scandinavia* 120: 441–445.

Belluck, P., and B. Carey. 2013. Psychiatry's guide is out of touch with science, experts say. *New York Times*, May 6.

Belmaker, R., and G. Agam. 2008. Major depressive disorder. *New England Journal of Medicine* 358: 55–68.

Benson, H., and M. Klipper. 2000. *The Relaxation Response*. Updated ed. New York: HarperCollins, 2000.

Bergner, Daniel. 2009. Women who want to want. *New York Times*, November 24.

Berk, M., S. Jeavons, O. Dean, et al. 2009. Nail-biting stuff? The effect of N-acetyl cysteine on nail biting. *CNS Spectrums* 14: 357–360.

Berne, Eric. 1964. *Games People Play*. New York: Grove Press.

Blashfield, R. 1998. Diagnostic models and systems. In *Clinical Psychology: Assessment*, ed. A. Bellack, M. Herson, and C. Reynolds, 4: 57–59. New York: Elsevier Science.

Blumentahl, James, Michael Babyak, Kathleen Moore, et al. 1999. Effects of exercise training on older adults with major depression. *Archives of Internal Medicine* 159: 2349–2356.

Bockoven, Sanbourne, and Harry Soloman. 1975. Comparison of two five-year follow-up studies: 1947 to 1952 and 1967 to 1972. *American Journal of Psychiatry* 132: 798–801.

Bonnie, Richard, John Jeffries, and Peter Low. 2000. *A Case Study in the Insanity Defense: The Trial of John W. Hinckley, Jr.* 2nd ed. New York: Foundation Press.

Bourne, Peter. 1971. *Men, Stress, and Viet Nam*. New York: Little Brown.

Brafman, Ori, and Rom Brafman. 2008. *Sway*. New York: Doubleday.

Breggin, Peter. 1991. *Toxic Psychiatry*. New York: St. Martin's Press.

———. 2008. *Medication Madness*. New York: St. Martin's Press.

Broocks, Andreas, Borwin Bandelow, Gunda Pekrun, et al. 1998. Comparison of aerobic exercise, clomipramine, and placebo in the treatment of panic disorder. *American Journal of Psychiatry* 155: 603–609.

Brownlee, Shannon. 2007. *Overtreated*. New York: Bloomsbury USA.

Buber, Martin. 1958. *I and Thou*. Trans. Ronald Gregor Smith. New York: Charles Scribner's Sons.

Buchanan, R. 2010. The 2009 PORT psychopharmacological treatment recommendations and summary statements. *Schizophrenia Bulletin* 36: 71–93.

Calton, T., M. Ferriter, N. Huband, et al. 2008. A systematic review of the Soteria paradigm for the treatment of people diagnosed with schizophrenia. *Schizophrenia Bulletin* 34: 181–192.

Carey, Benedict. 2006. Revisiting schizophrenia: Are drugs always needed? *New York Times*, March 21.

———. 2010a. In cybertherapy, avatars assist with healing. *New York Times*, November 22.

————. 2010b. Revising book on disorders of the mind. *New York Times*, February 10.

————. 2011. Drugs used for psychosis go to youths in foster care. *New York Times*, November 21.

Carey, Benedict, and Harris Gardiner. 2008. Psychiatric group faces scrutiny over drug industry ties. *New York Times*, July 12.

Carey, Benedict, and John Markoff. 2010. Students, meet your new teacher, Mr. Robot. *New York Times*, July 11.

Carlat, Daniel. 2009. Pristiq: An update. *Carlat Psychiatry Report* 7: 3–6.

————. 2010. *Unhinged: The Trouble with Psychiatry–A Doctor's Revelations about a Profession in Crisis*. New York: Free Press.

————. 2010. Mind over meds: How I decided my psychiatry patients needed more from me than prescriptions. *New York Times Magazine* (April 25): 41–43.

Carney, Caroline, Laura Jones, and Robert Woolson. 2006. Medical comorbidity in women and men with schizophrenia. *Journal of General Internal Medicine* 21: 1133–1137.

Cassell, Eric. 1979. *The Healer's Art*. New York: Penguin Books.

Cattell, Heather. 1989. *The 16 PF: Personality in Depth*. Champaign, IL: Institute for Personality and Ability Testing.

CBS News. 2012. Treating depression: Is there a placebo effect? *CBS 60 Minutes*, February 18.

Cheung, V., C. Chiu, C. Law, et al. 2011. Positive symptoms and white matter microstructure in never-medicated first episode schizophrenia. *Psychological Medicine* 41: 1709–1719.

Chochinov, H., T. Hack, T. Hassard, et al. 2005. Dignity therapy: A novel psychotherapeutic intervention for patients near the end of life. *Journal of Clinical Oncology* 23: 5520–5525.

Chouinard, Guy. 1980. Neuroleptic-induced supersensitivity psychosis: Clinical and pharmacological characteristics. *American Journal of Psychiatry* 137: 16–20.

Ciompi, L. 1980. Catamestic long-term study on the course of life and aging of schizophrenics. *Schizophrenia Bulletin* 6: 606–618.

Ciompi, H., P. Dauwalder, and C. Maier. 1992. The pilot project 'Soteria Berne': Clinical experiences and results. *British Journal of Psychiatry* 161: 145–153.

Climo, Lawrence. 2009. *Psychiatrist on the Road*. Point Richmond, CA: Bay Tree Publishing.

Cocozza, Joseph, and Henry Steadman. 1976. The failure of psychiatric predictions of dangerous: Clear and convincing evidence. *Rutgers Law Review* 29: 1084–1101.

Colton, Tim, Michael Ferriter, Nick Huband, et al. 2008. A systematic review of the Soteria paradigm for the treatment of people diagnosed with schizophrenia. *Schizophrenia Bulletin* 34: 181–192.

Cooper, Richard. 2003. Where is psychiatry going and who is going there? *Academic Psychiatry* 27: 229–234.

Coppen, A., and J. Bailey. 2000. Enhancement of the antidepressant action of fluoxetine by folic acid: A randomized, placebo controlled trial. *Journal of Affective Disorders* 60: 121–130.

Correll, C., P. Manu, V. Olshansky, et al. 2009. Cardiometabolic risk of second-generation antipsychotic medications during first-time use in children and adolescents. *Journal of the American Medical Association* 302: 1765–1773.

Cosgrove, Lisa, Sheldon Krimsky, Manisha Vijayaraghavan, et al. 2006. Financial ties between *DSM-IV* panel members and the pharmaceutical industry. *Psychotherapy and Psychosomatics* 75: 154–160.

Crawford, M. 2000. Homicide is impossible to predict. *Psychiatric Bulletin* 24: 152.

Dao, James. 2012. Branding a soldier with "personality disorder." *New York Times*, February 25.

Davies, James. 2013. *Cracked: The Unhappy Truth about Psychiatry*. New York: Penguin Books.

Davis, J., W. Giakas, J. Qu, et al. 2011. Should we treat depression with drugs or psychological interventions? *Philosophy, Ethics, and Humanities in Medicine* 6: 8.

deMaat, S., J. Dekker, R. Schoevers, et al. 2006. Relative efficacy of psychotherapy and psychopharmacology in the treatment of depression: A meta-analysis. *Psychotherapy Research* 16: 562–572.

Dewan, Mantosh. 1999. Are psychiatrists cost-effective? An analysis of integrated versus split treatment. *American Journal of Psychiatry* 156: 324–326.

Difede, J., J. Cukor, N. Jayasinghe, et al. 1995. Virtual reality exposure therapy for the treatment of post-traumatic stress disorder following September 11, 2001. *American Journal of Psychiatry* 68: 1639–1647.

Druss, Benjamin, Silke Esenwein, Michael Compton, et al. 2010. A randomized trial of medical care management for community mental health settings: The primary care access, referral, and evaluation (PCARE) study. *American Journal of Psychiatry* 167: 151–159.

Druss, Benjamin, Steven Marcus, Jeannie Campbell, et al. 2008. Medical services for clients in community mental health centers: Results from a national survey. *Psychiatric Services* 59: 917–920.

Eby, George. 2006. Rapid recovery from major depression using magnesium treatment. *Medical Hypothesis* 67: 362–370.

Economist staff writer. 2013. Shrink wrapping: A single book has come to dominate psychiatry. *Economist*, May 18.

Engel, George. 1977. The need for a new medical model: A challenge for biomedicine. *Science* 196: 129–136.

Erickson, K., and A. Dramer. 2009. Aerobic exercise effects on cognitive and neural plasticity in older adults. *British Journal of Sports Medicine* 43: 22–24.

Etminan, M., F. Mikelberg, and J. Brophy. 2010. Selective serotonin reuptake inhibitors and the risk of cataracts: A nested case-control study. *Ophthalmology* 117: 1251–1255.

Everson, S., D. Goldberg, and G. Kaplan. 1996. Hopelessness and risk of mortality. *Psychosomatic Medicine* 58: 112–121.

Fawcett, Jan. 2010. Child psychopharmacology comes of age. *Psychiatric Annals* 40: 178.

Festinger, Leon. 1957. *A Theory of Cognitive Dissonance*. Stanford, CA: Stanford University Press.

Fisher, M., C. Holland, M. Marzenich, et al. 2009. Using neuroplasticity-based auditory training to improve verbal memory in schizophrenia. *American Journal of Psychiatry* 166: 805–811.

Fogelson, David. 2010. What's new in psychopharmacology: Controversies, breakthroughs, and tips. *Psychiatric Times* 27 (4).

Fournier, J., R. DeRubeis, S. Hollon, et al. 2010. Antidepressant drug effects and depression severity: A patient-level meta-analysis. *Journal of the American Medical Association* 303: 47–53.

Frances, Allen. 2010. A warning sign on the road to *DSM-V*: Beware of its unintended consequences. *Psychiatric Times* 26 (8)

———. 2012. Diagnosing the *DSM*. *New York Times*, May 12.

Frank, Jerome, and Julia Frank. 1991. *Persuasion and Healing: A Comparative Study of Psychotherapy*. 3rd ed. Baltimore: John Hopkins University Press.

Friedman, Richard. 2006. Violence and mental illness—how strong is the link? *New England Journal of Medicine* 355: 2064–2066.

Gardos, George, and Jonathan Cole. 1976. Maintenance antipsychotic therapy: Is the cure worse than the disease? *American Journal of Psychiatry* 133: 32–36.

George, Mark, Sarah Lisanby, David Avery, et al. 2010. Daily left prefrontal transcranial magnetic stimulation therapy for major depressive disorder. *Archives of General Psychiatry* 67: 507–516.

Gillman, P. 2013. Atypical antipsychotics: Where is the science, where is the evidence? *The Carlat Report (Psychiatry)* 11 (1): 1, 3, 5–8.

Gordon, C., and M. Green. 2013. Shared decision making in the treatment of psychosis. *Psychiatric Times* 30 (4).

Grant, J., S. Kim, and B. Odlaug. 2007. N-acetyl cysteine, a glutamate-modulating agent, in the treatment of pathological gambling: A pilot study. *Biological Psychiatry* 62: 652–657.

Grant, J., B. Odlaug, and S. Kim. 2009. N-acetylcysteine, a glutamate modulator, in the treatment of trichotillomania. *Archives of General Psychiatry* 66: 756–763.

Greenberg, Gary. 2013. *The Book of Woe: The DSM and the Unmasking of Psychiatry*. New York: Blue Rider Press.

Greenberg, Stuart, and Daniel Shuman. 1997. Irreconcilable conflict between therapeutic and forensic roles. *Professional Psychology: Research and Practice* 28: 50–57.

Haley, Jay. 1990. *Strategies of Psychotherapy.* 2nd ed. Williston, VT: Crown Publishing.

Harding, Courtenay. 1988. Course types in schizophrenia: An analysis of European and American studies. *Schizophrenia Bulletin* 14: 633–643.

Harding, Courtenay, and James Zahniser. 1994. Empirical correction of seven myths about schizophrenia with implications for treatment. *ACTA Psychiatrica Scandinavia* 90 (supplement 384): 140–146.

Harris, Gardiner. 2011a. Antipsychotic drugs called hazardous for the elderly. *New York Times*, May 9.

———. 2011b. Talk doesn't pay, so psychiatry turns to drug therapy. *New York Times*, March 5.

Harrow, M., T. Jobe, and R. Faull. 2012. Do all schizophrenia patients need antipsychotic treatment continuously throughout their lifetime? A 20-year longitudinal study. *Psychological Medicine* 42: 2145–2155.

Ho, B., N. Andreasen, S. Ziebell, et al. 2011. Long-term antipsychotic treatment and brain volumes: A longitudinal study of first-episode schizophrenia. *Archives of General Psychiatry* 68: 128–137.

Horgan, John. 1999. *The Undiscovered Mind: How the Brain Defies Replication, Medication, and Explanation.* New York: Free Press.

House, James, Karl Landis, and Debra Umberson. 1988. Social relationships and health. *Science* 241: 540–545.

Hua, J., P. Shih, S. Golshan, et al. 2012. Comparison of longer-term safety and effectiveness of 4 atypical antipsychotics in patients over age 40: A trial using equipoise-stratified randomization. *Journal of Clinical Psychiatry* (online ahead of print). November 27. www.psychiatrist.com.

Hyman, Steven. 2003. What are the right targets for psychopharmacology? *Science* 299: 349–350.

Insel, Thomas. 2009. Translating scientific opportunity into public health impact: A strategic plan for research on mental illness. *Archives of General Psychiatry* 66: 128–133.

Jamison, Kay. 1995. *An Unquiet Mind: A Memoir of Moods and Madness.* New York: Alfred A. Knopf.

Jazayeri, S., M. Tehrani-Doost, S. Keshavarz, et al. 2008. Comparison of therapeutic effects of omega-3 fatty acid eicosapentaenoic acid and fluoxetine, separately and in combination, in major depressive disorder. *Australia New Zealand Journal of Psychiatry* 42: 192–198.

Kabat-Zinn, J., A. Massion, J. Kristeller, et al. 1992. Effectiveness of a meditation-based stress reduction program in the treatment of anxiety disorders. *American Journal of Psychiatry* 149: 936–943.

Kagan, J., and N. Snidman. 2004. *The Long Shadow of Temperament*. Cambridge, MA: Harvard University Press.

Kandel, Eric. 1998. A new intellectual framework for psychiatry. *American Journal of Psychiatry* 155: 457–468.

Kane, John. 2010. Maintenance strategies in schizophrenia. *CNS Spectrums* 15 (4) Supplement 6: 12–14.

Kaplan, K., D. Goldenberg, and M. Galvin-Nadeau. 1993. The impact of a meditation-based stress reduction program on fibromyalgia. *General Hospital Psychiatry* 15: 284–289.

Kelly, George. 1963. *A Theory of Personality: The Psychology of Personal Constructs*. New York: W. W. Norton.

Kelly, Janis. 2009. Psychiatrists urged to help the mentally ill stop smoking. *Medscape Medical News*, September 21 (online).

Khan, Aman. 1999. How do psychotropic medications really work? *Psychiatric Times* 16 (10).

Kim, I., L. Gylm, C. Schetter, et al. 2009. Risk of post partum depressive symptoms with elevated corticotrophin-releasing hormone in human pregnancy. *Archives of General Psychiatry* 66: 162–169.

Kirsch, Irving. 2009. *The Emperor's New Drugs: Exploding the Antidepressant Myth*. London: Bodley Head.

Kirsch, Irving, Thomas Moore, Alan Scoboria, et al. 2002. The emperor's new drugs: An analysis of antidepressant medication data submitted to the U.S. Food and Drug Administration. *Prevention & Treatment* 5, article 23.

Kleinman, Arthur. 1988. *Rethinking Psychiatry*. New York: Free Press.

Kocsis, J., R. Friedman, J. Markowitz, et al. 1996. Maintenance therapy for chronic depression. *Archives of General Psychiatry* 53: 769–774.

Konstantinidou, Charitomeni, and Luiz Dratcu. 2006. The use of physical exercise in psychiatry: Prescribing aerobic exercise in panic disorder. *Annals of General Psychiatry* 5 (Supplement 1): S25.

Koran, Lorrin, E. Aboujaoude, and N. Gamel. 2009. Double-blind study of dextroamphetamine versus caffeine augmentation for treatment-resistant obsessive-compulsive disorder. *Journal of Clinical Psychiatry* 70: 1530–1535.

Koran, Lorrin, H. Sox, K. Marton, et al. 1989. Medical evaluation of psychiatric patients: 1. Results in a state mental health system. *Archives of General Psychiatry* 46: 733–740.

Kramer, Peter. 1993. *Listening to Prozac*. New York: Penguin Group.

Laaksonen, D., H. Lakka, L. Niskanen, et al. 2002. Metabolic syndrome and development of diabetes mellitus: Application and validation of recently suggested definitions of metabolic syndrome in a prospective cohort study. *American Journal of Epidemiology* 156: 1070–1077.

Laan, W., D. Grubber, J-P Shelten, et al. 2010, Adjuvant aspirin therapy reduces symptoms of schizophrenia spectrum disorders: Results from a randomized double-blind, placebo-controlled trial. *Journal of Clinical Psychiatry* 71: 520–527.

Lake, James, and David Spiegel, eds. 2007. *Complementary and Alternative Treatments in Mental Health Care.* Arlington, VA: American Psychiatric Publishing.

Lanier, Jaron. 2010. On the threshold of the avatar era. *Wall Street Journal*, October 23–24, C3.

LaRowe, Steven, Hugh Myrick, Sarra Hedden, et al. 2007. Is cocaine desire reduced by N-acetylcysteine? *American Journal of Psychiatry* 164: 1115–1117.

Leucht, S., M. Tardy, and K. Komossa. 2012. Antipsychotic drugs versus placebo for relapse prevention in schizophrenia: A systematic review and meta-analysis. *Lancet* 371: 2063–2071.

Levine, J. 1997. Controlled trials of inositol in psychiatry. *European Neuropsychopharmacology* 7: 147–155.

Lieberman, Jeffrey, Scott Stroup, Joseph McEvoy, et al. 2005. Effectiveness of antipsychotic drugs in patients with chronic schizophrenia. *New England Journal of Medicine* 353: 1209–1223.

Lilienfeld, Scott, Lynn Ruscio, John Ruscio, et al. 2010. The top ten myths of popular psychology. *Skeptic Magazine* 15: 36–41.

Linden, David. 2011. *The Compass of Pleasure.* New York: Penguin Group (Viking).

Lipovac, Markus. 2010. Improvement of postmenopausal depressive and anxiety symptoms after treatment with isoflavones derived from red clover extracts. *Maturitas* 65: 258–261.

Lucas, M., F. Mirzaei, A. Pan, et al. 2011. Coffee, caffeine, and risk of depression among women. *Archives of Internal Medicine* 171: 1571–1578.

Luhrmann, T. 2013. The violence in our heads. *New York Times*, September 19.

Makris, N., L. Seidman, T. Ahern, et al. 2010. White matter volume abnormalities and associations with symptomatology in schizophrenia. *Psychiatry Research: Neuroimaging* 183: 21–29.

Marinoff, Lou. 1999. *Plato Not Prozac!* New York: NJF Books.

Martin, Douglas. 2010. Harriet Shetler, 92; helped to found mental illness group. *New York Times* (Obituaries), April 4.

McAdams, Dan. 1993. *The Stories We Live By.* New York: Guilford Press.

McHugh, Paul. 2006. *The Mind Has Mountains.* Baltimore: Johns Hopkins University Press.

———. 2013. A manual run amok. *Wall Street Journal*, May 18/19.

McHugh, Paul, and Phillip Slavney. 1998. *The Perspectives of Psychiatry*. 2nd ed. Baltimore: Johns Hopkins University Press.

McKee, Robert. 1997. *Story*. New York: Regan Books.

Meltzer, Herbert, and William Bobo. 2006. Interpreting the efficacy findings in the CATIE study: What clinicians should know. *CNS Spectrums* 11 (7), Supplement 7: 14–24.

Meyers, Isabel Briggs, and Peter Meyers. 1980. *Gifts Differing: Understanding Personality Type*. Mountain View, CA: Davies-Black Publishing.

Miller, A., V. Maletic, and C. Raison. 2009. Inflammation and its discontents: The role of cytokines in the pathophysiology of major depression. *Biological Psychiatry* 65: 732–741.

Mischoulon, D., G. Papakostas, and C. Dording. 2009. A double-blind, randomized controlled trial of ethyl-eicosapentaenoate for major depression. *Journal of Clinical Psychiatry* 70: 1636–1644.

Miyaoka, T., R. Yasukawa, H. Yasuda, et al. 2007. Possible antipsychotic effects of minocycline in patients with schizophrenia. *Progress in Neuro-Psychopharmacological Biological Psychiatry* 31: 304–307.

———. 2008. Minocycline as adjunctive therapy for schizophrenia: An open-label study. *Clinical Neuropharmacology* 31: 287–292.

Moffic, H. S. 2012. How to end a psychiatric epidemic: Whitaker's warning, Wallace's wisdom—and the redemption of psychiatry. *Psychiatric Times* 29 (8): 10–11.

Molina, Brooke, Stephen Hinshaw, James Swanson, et al. 2009. The MTA at 8 years: Prospective follow-up of children treated for combined-type ADHD in a multisite study. *Journal of the Academy of Child and Adolescent Psychiatry* 48: 484–500.

Monahan, J. 1997. Actuarial support for the clinical assessment of violence risk. *International Review of Psychiatry* 9: 167–170.

Moncrieff, J., S. Wessely, and R. Hardy. 2012. Tricyclic antidepressants compared with active placebos for depression. *Cochrane Summaries*. www.searchmedica.com. October 17.

Moore, David, and Jim Corbett. 2012. Adderall stirs strong emotions. *New York Times*, November 28.

Morisano, D., I. Bacher, J. Audrain-McGovern, et al. 2009. Mechanisms underlying the comorbidity of tobacco use in mental health and addictive disorders. *Canadian Journal of Psychiatry* 54: 356–367.

Mosher, Loren. 1978. Community residential treatment for schizophrenia: Two-year follow up. *Hospital and Community Psychiatry* 29: 715–723.

Muller, René. 2008. *Doing Psychiatry Wrong: A Critical and Prescriptive Look at a Faltering Profession*. New York: Analytic Press/Taylor & Francis Group.

Nasrallah, Henry. 2010. A psychiatric manifesto. *Current Psychiatry* 9 (4): 7–8.

————. 2012. Why are metabolic monitoring guidelines being ignored? *Current Psychiatry* 11 (12): 4–5.

Nemets, H., B. Nemets, A. Apter, et al. 2006. Omega-3 treatment of childhood depression: A controlled, double-blind pilot study. *American Journal of Psychiatry* 163: 1098–1100.

Nestler, Eric, and Steven Hyman. 2010. Animal models of neuropsychiatric disorders. *Nature Neuroscience* 13: 1161–1169.

New York Times Editorial Board. 2013. Shortcomings of a psychiatric Bible. *New York Times*, May 11.

Nicks, Stevie. 2011. My favorite mistake. *Newsweek*, May 1.

Nigg, Joel. 2009. Cognitive impairments found with attention-deficit/hyperactivity disorder. *Psychiatric Times* 26 (3).

NIMH 2006. Questions and answers about the NIMH sequenced treatment alternatives to relieve depression (STAR* D) study—all medication levels. November. www.nimh.nih.gov/healthtrials.

Oldham, J., D. Carlat, R. Friedman, and M. Nierenberg. 2011. Angell, "The illusions of psychiatry": An exchange. *New York Review of Books*, August 18.

Oldham, John, and Lois Morris. 1990. *Personality Self-Portrait*. New York: Bantam Books.

Olfson, Mark. 2010. Antipsychotics for children: What we know—what we need to know. *Psychiatric Times* 27 (2).

Olfson, M., S. Crystal, C. Huang, et al. 2010. Trends in antipsychotic drug use by very young, privately insured children. *Journal of the American Academy of Child and Adolescent Psychiatry* 49: 3–6.

Ongur, D. 2009. Topics in the treatments of schizophrenia. *The Carlat Psychiatry Report* 7 (12): 4.

Pan, An, M. Lucas, R. van Dam, et al. 2010. Bidirectional association between depression and type 2 diabetes mellitus in women. *Archives of Internal Medicine* 170: 1876–1883.

Papakostas, G., C. Cassiello, and N. Iuvieno. 2012. Folates and s-adenosylmethionine for major depressive disorder. *Canadian Journal of Psychiatry* 57: 406–413.

Papakostas, G., D. Mischoulon, I. Shyu, et al. 2010. S-adenosylmethionine (SAMe) augmentation of serotonin reuptake inhibitors for antidepressant nonresponders with major depressive disorder: A double-blind, randomized clinical trial. *American Journal of Psychiatry* 167: 942–948.

Parks, Joseph. 2008. Overview: The problem. *Psychiatric Times* 25 (Supplement), December.

Patterson, C. 1984. Empathy, warmth, and genuineness in psychotherapy: A review of reviews. *Psychotherapy* 21: 431–438.

Peet, M. 2001. Two double-blind placebo-controlled pilot studies of eicosapentaenoic acid in the treatment of schizophrenia. *Schizophrenia Research* 49: 243–251.

Perkins, Diana, Hongbin Gu, Kalina Boteva, et al. 2005. Relationship between duration of untreated psychosis and outcome in first-episode schizophrenia: A critical review and meta-analysis. *American Journal of Psychiatry* 162: 1785–1804.

Pink, Daniel. 2005. *A Whole New Mind*. New York: Riverhead Books.

Poeldinger, W. 1991. A functional-dimensional approach to depression: Serotonin deficiency as a target syndrome in a comparison of 5-hydroxytryptophan and fluvoxamine. *Psychopathology* 24: 53–81.

Pomeroy, Claire, James Mitchell, James Roerig, et al. 2002. *Medical Complications of Psychiatric Illness*. Washington, DC: American Psychiatric Publishing.

Porizkova, Paulina. 2011. Ending a midlife affair with meds. *Huffington Post*, May 18 (online).

Poulton, Alison. 2006. Long-term outcomes of stimulant medication in attention-deficit hyperactivity disorder. *Expert Review of Neurotherapeutics* 6 (4): 551–561.

Price, Lawrence. 2011. Antipsychotics and brain volume reductions in schizophrenia patients. *Brown University Psychopharmacology Update* 22 (5): 1, 5–6.

Rappaport, Maurice. 1978. Are there schizophrenics for whom drugs may be unnecessary or contraindicated? *International Pharmacopsychiatry* 13: 100–111.

Ratey, John, with Eric Hagerman. 2008. *Spark: The Revolutionary New Science of Exercise and the Brain*. New York: Little, Brown.

Richo, David. 2006. *The Five Things We Cannot Change*. Boston: Shambhala Publications.

Risch, S., and C. Nemeroff. 1992. Neurochemical alterations of serotonergic neuronal systems in depression. *Journal of Clinical Psychiatry* 53: 3–7.

Riso, Richard, and Russ Hudson. 1999. *The Wisdom of the Enneagram*. New York: Bantam Books.

Rochon, P., S. Normand, T. Gomes, et al. 2008. Antipsychotic therapy and short-term serious events in older adults with dementia. *Archives of Internal Medicine* 168: 1090–1096.

Rosenhan, David. 1973. On being sane in insane places. *Science* 179: 250–258.

Rothbaum, B., L. Hodges, S. Smith, et al. 2000. A controlled study of virtual reality exposure therapy for the fear of flying. *Journal of Consultation and Clinical Psychology* 68: 1020–1026.

Sacks, Oliver. 2010. *The Mind's Eye*. New York: Alfred A. Knopf.

Saks, Elyn. 2007. *The Center Cannot Hold: My Journey Through Madness*. New York: Hyperion.

Sapolsky, Robert. 2004. *Why Zebras Don't Get Ulcers*. 3rd ed. New York: Henry Holt and Company.

Schmidt, Peter, Robert Daly, Miki Bloch, et al. 2005. Dehydroepiandrosterone monotherapy in midlife-onset major and minor depression. *Archives of General Psychiatry* 62: 154–162.

Schneider, R., C. Alexander, F. Staggers, et al. 2005. Long-term effects of stress reduction on mortality in persons > 55 years of age with systemic hypertension. *American Journal of Cardiology* 95: 1060–1064.

Schooler, Nina. 1967. One year after discharge: Community adjustment of schizophrenia patients. *American Journal of Psychiatry* 123: 986–995.

Schwarz, Alan. 2012. Drowned in a stream of prescriptions. *New York Times*, January 1.

———. 2013. Attention-deficit drugs face new campus rules. *New York Times*, April 30.

Schwarz, Alan, and Sarah Cohen. 2013. More diagnoses of hyperactivity in new C.D.C. data. *New York Times*, March 31.

Science Illustrated. 2010. The brain explorers. March–April.

Scott, C., and P. Resnick. 2002. Assessing risk of violence in psychiatric patients. *Psychiatric Times* 19 (4) Special report: forensic psychiatry.

Scott, Charles. 2005. Overview of the criminal justice system. In *Handbook of Correctional Mental Health*, ed. Charles Scott and Joan Gerbasi. Washington, DC: American Psychiatric Publishing.

Seligman, Martin. 1975. *Helplessness: On Depression, Development, and Death*. San Francisco: W. H. Freeman.

Shapiro, Arthur, and Elaine Shapiro. 1997. *The Powerful Placebo*. Baltimore: Johns Hopkins University Press.

Shea, Jack. 2012. Fox8 TV, Akron, Ohio, February 13.

Shenk, Joshua. 2009. What makes us happy? *Atlantic Monthly*, June, 36–53.

Shorter, Edward. 2009. *Before Prozac: The Troubled History of Mood Disorders*. New York: Oxford University Press.

Siegal, Daniel. 2010. *Mindsight: The New Science of Personal Transformation*. New York: Random House.

Soczynska, J., L. Zhang, S. Kennedy, et al. 2012. Are psychiatric disorders inflammatory-based conditions? *Psychiatric Times* 29 (10): 24–25.

Sokal, J., E. Messias, F. Dickerson, et al. 2004. Comorbidity of medical illnesses among adults with serious mental illness who are receiving community psychiatric services. *Journal of Nervous and Mental Diseases* 192: 421–427.

Solomon, Andrew. 2001. *The Noonday Demon*. New York: Scribner.

Spek, V., P. Cuijpers, I. Nyklicek, et al. 2007. Internet-based cognitive behavior therapy for symptoms of depression and anxiety: A meta-analysis. *Psychological Medicine* 37: 319–328.

Spitzer, R., and J. Fleiss. 1974. A re-analysis of the reliability of psychiatric diagnoses. *British Journal of Psychiatry* 125: 341–347.

Sroufe, L. 2012. Ritalin gone wrong. *New York Times* (Sunday Review), January 29, 1, 6.

Stahl, Stephen. 2010. Enhancing outcome from major depression: Using antidepressant combination therapies with multifunctional pharmacologic mechanisms from the initiation of treatment. *CNS Spectrums* 15 (2): 79–94.

Steadman, H., A. Redlich, L. Callahan, et al. 2010. Effect of mental health courts on arrests and jail days. *Archives of General Psychiatry* (online), October 4.

Studd, J. 2012. Severe premenstrual syndrome and bipolar disorder: A tragic confusion. *Menopause International* 18: 82–86.

Styron, William. 1990. *Darkness Visible: A Memoir of Madness*. New York: Vintage Books.

Su, K.-P., S.-Y. Huang, C.-C. Chiu, et al. 2003. Omega-3 fatty acids in major depressive disorder: A preliminary double-blind, placebo-controlled trial. *European Neuropsychopharmacology* 13: 267–271.

Swartz, Marvin, Scott Stroup, Joseph McEvoy, et al. 2008. What CATIE found: Results from the schizophrenia trial. *Psychiatric Services* 59: 500–506.

Szasz, Thomas. 1961. *The Myth of Mental Illness: Foundations of a Theory of Personal Conduct*. New York: Hoeber-Harper.

Szmukler, G. 2001. Violence prediction in practice. *British Journal of Psychiatry* 178: 84–85.

Tavris, Carol. 2013. How psychiatry went crazy. *Wall Street Journal*, May 17.

Taylor, Daniel. 1996. *The Healing Power of Stories*. New York: Doubleday.

Taylor, Robert. 1982. *Mind or Body: Distinguishing Psychological from Organic Disorders*. New York: McGraw-Hill Book Company.

———. 1990. *Health Fact, Health Fiction*. Dallas: Taylor Publishing Company.

———. 2007. *Psychological Masquerade: Distinguishing Psychological from Organic Disorders*. 3rd ed. New York: Springer Publishing Company.

Taylor, Robert, and E. Fuller Torrey. 1972. The self-education of psychiatric residents. *American Journal of Psychiatry* 128: 1116–1121.

TED. 2013. Today's TED talk, Derek Paravicini and Adam Ockelford: In the key of genius. August 9.

Tenzel, James, and Robert Taylor. 1969. An evaluation of hypnosis and suggestion as treatment for warts. *Psychosomatics* 10: 252–257.

Thomas, A., S. Chess, and H. Birch. 1970. The origin of personality. *Scientific American* 223: 102–109.

Thomas, M., W. Dong, and J. Jankovic. 2003. Minocycline and other tetracycline derivatives: A neuroprotective strategy in Parkinson's disease and Huntington's disease. *Clinical Neuropharmacology* 26: 18–23.

Thomas, Rosanne, and Daniel Peterson. 2003. A neurogenic theory of depression gains momentum. *Molecular Interventions* 3: 441–444.

Torrey, Fuller. 1974. *The Death of Psychiatry*. Radnor, PA: Chilton Book Company.

———. 2013. Treat the 1 percent. *National Review* 65 (January 28): 26, 28.

———. 2014. *American Psychosis*. New York: Oxford University Press.

Torrey, Fuller, Aaron Kennard, Don Eslinger, et al. 2010. More mentally ill persons are in jails and prisons than hospitals: A survey of the states. Treatment Advocacy Center (news release). Arlington, VA, May 12.

Torrey, Fuller, and M. Peterson. 1973. Slow and latent viruses in schizophrenia. *Lancet* 302: 22–24.

Torrey, Fuller, Jonathan Stanley, and John Monahan. 2008. The MacArthur violence risk assessment study revisited: Two views ten years after its initial publication. *Psychiatric Services* 59: 147–152.

Tucker, Gary. 1998. Putting *DSM-IV* in perspective. *American Journal of Psychiatry* 155: 159–161.

Tucker, William. 2007. *How People Change: The Short Story as Case History*. New York: Other Press.

Turkewitz, J., and L. Linderman. 2012. The disability trap. *New York Times*, October 21.

Turner, E., A. Matthews, E. Linardatos, et al. 2008. Selective publication of antidepressant trials and its influence on apparent efficacy. *New England Journal of Medicine* 358: 252–260.

Verweij, Karin, Brendan Zietsch, Sarah Medland, et al. 2010. A genome-wide association study of Cloninger's temperament scales: Implications for the evolutionary genetics of personality. *Biological Psychology* 85: 306–317.

Viguera, A., R. Baldessarini, J. Hegarty, et al. 1997. Clinical risk following abrupt and gradual withdrawal. *Archives of General Psychiatry* 54: 49–55.

Villeneuve, K., S. Potvin, and N. Lesage. 2010. Meta-analysis of rates of drop-out from psychosocial treatment among persons with schizophrenia spectrum disorder. *Schizophrenia Research* 121: 266–270.

Vonnegut, Mark. 1975. *The Eden Express: A Memoir of Insanity*. New York: Seven Stories Press.

Wallace, Robert, and Herbert Benson. 1972. The physiology of meditation. *Scientific American* 226: 84–90.

Warner, Richard. 1987. *Recovery from Schizophrenia: Psychiatry and Political Economy*. New York: Routledge & Kegan Paul.

Watters, Ethan. 2010. *Crazy Like Us: The Globalization of the American Psyche*. New York: Free Press.

Whitaker, Robert. 2002. *Mad in America*. Cambridge, MA: Perseus Publishing.

———. 2010. *Anatomy of an Epidemic*. New York: Crown Publishers.

Wigner, Eugene. 1969. Are we machines? *Proceedings of the American Philosophical Society* 113: 95–101.

Wilson, Duff. 2009. Weight gain associated with antipsychotics. *New York Times*, October 27.

————. 2010. Child's ordeal shows risks of psychosis drugs for young. *New York Times*, September 1.

Winslade, William, and Judith Ross. 1983. *The Insanity Plea: The Uses and Abuses of the Insanity Defense*. New York: Charles Scribner's Sons.

Wolkowitz, Owen, Victor Reus, Audrey Keebler, et al. 1999. Double-blind treatment of major depression with dehydroepiandrosterone. *American Journal of Psychiatry* 156: 646–649.

Wright, P., M. Birkett, and S. David. 2001. Double-blind placebo controlled comparison of intramuscular olanzapine and intramuscular haloperidol in the treatment of acute agitation in schizophrenia. *American Journal of Psychiatry* 158: 1149–1151.

Wu, J., A. Yeung, R. Schnyer, et al. 2012. Acupuncture for depression: A review of clinical applications. *Canadian Journal of Psychiatry* 57: 397–405.

Wunderink, L., R. Nieboer, D. Wiersman, et al. 2013. Recovery in remitted first-episode psychosis at 7 years of follow-up of an early dose reduction/discontinuation or maintenance treatment strategy: Long-term follow-up of a 2-year randomized clinical trial. *JAMA Psychiatry* 70: 913–920.

Wyatt, Richard. 1991. Neuroleptics and the natural course of schizophrenia. *Schizophrenia Bulletin* 17: 325–351.

Wyden, Peter. 1998. *Conquering Schizophrenia: A Father, His Son, and a Medical Breakthrough*. New York: Alfred A. Knopf.

Yalom, Irvin. 2002. *The Gift of Therapy*. New York: Harper Perennial.

Yim, I., L. Glynn, P. Shetler, et al. 2009. Risk of postpartum depressive symptoms with elevated corticotrophin-releasing hormone in human pregnancy. *Archives of General Psychiatry* 66: 162–169.

Yohannes, Mengistu, and Robert Baldwin. 2008. Medical comorbitities in late-life depression. *Psychiatric Times* 25 (14).

Yung, A., H. Yuen, G. Berger, et al. 2007. Declining transition rate in ultra high risk (prodromal) services: Dilution or reduction of risk? *Schizophrenia Bulletin* 33: 675–681.

INDEX

191

ABOUT THE AUTHOR

Trained in psychiatry at Stanford University School of Medicine, Dr. Robert Taylor spent his early career designing and managing mental health programs, consulting, and teaching. A training specialist in the Psychiatry Training Branch at the National Institute of Mental Health, he consulted with the United States Secret Service on presidential assassination, testified before Congress on national health insurance, and helped start a free clinic in Bethesda, Maryland. In the early 1970s he directed community mental health services in Marin County, California, and then for eight years worked as a consulting psychiatrist to the state of California on wellness promotion. For several years he lectured at Stanford as clinical associate professor of medicine. Later still, he directed student health services at California State University, Northridge, before moving on to serve as medical director of community mental health services and a private psychiatric hospital in Austin, Texas. Most recently, Dr. Taylor has practiced clinical psychiatry in New Zealand, Alaska, Texas, Idaho, Montana, and California. In addition to numerous professional articles, he has authored *Mind or Body* (1982), *Health Fact, Health Fiction* (1990), and *Psychological Masquerade*, 3rd edition (2007).